Volume Replacement

Springer

Berlin
Heidelberg
New York
Barcelona
Budapest
Hong Kong
London
Milan
Paris
Santa Clara
Singapore
Tokyo

J.-F. Baron   J. Treib (Eds.)

Volume Replacement

Mit 23 Abbildungen

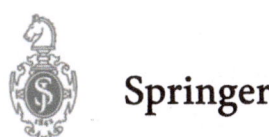 Springer

Professor Dr. med. JEAN-FRANCOIS BARON
Université Pierre
et Marie Curie Paris VI
Anesthesie-Reanimation
96, rue Didot
75014 Paris, France

Priv.-Doz. Dr. med. JOHANNES TREIB
Universitätskliniken des Saarlandes
Neurologische Klinik
Kirrbergerstraße
66421 Homburg/Saar, Germany

ISBN-13: 978-3-540-64187-2   e-ISBN-13: 978-3-642-72170-0
DOI: 10.1007/978-3-642-72170-0

CIP Data applied for
Die Deutsche Bibliothek – CIP-Einheitsaufnahme
Volume replacement / J.-F. Baron, J. Treib (ed.). – Berlin; Heidelberg; New York; Barcelona; Budapest; Hong Kong; London; Milan; Paris; Santa Clara; Singapore; Tokyo: Springer, 1998

Typesetting: K+V Fotosatz GmbH, Beerfelden
Cover-design: D & P, Heidelberg

SPIN 10652825   18/3137-5 4 3 2 1 0 – Printed on acid-free paper

Preface

Since the 1980s, the clinical practice of plasma volume expansion has changed considerably: fresh frozen plasma has been replaced by colloids. At the beginning of the 1990s, the administration of serum albumin was the most common means of plasma volume expansion, but it was misused in many clinical situations. Because albumin is sometimes in short supply and is currently more costly than artificial colloids, control of its overuse has significant clinical and economic ramifications for hospitals. In an effort to optimize the use of albumin, several societies of anesthesiologists and intensive care physicians have developed guidelines based on the currently available literature, demonstrating therapeutic equivalence between artificial colloids and albumin in many clinical situations. The impact of these guidelines has been a subject of debate since observational studies were conducted to characterize the use of albumin and artificial colloids and to determine the appropriateness of their use in accordance with the indication guidelines. In these studies, albumin is still frequently administered in surgical and critically ill patients, especially in intensive care settings, showing that albumin is often administered instead of artificial colloids. This discrepancy between the guidelines and common practice may reflect a lack of knowledge that albumin and artificial colloids are equally effective or a concern about the safety of artifical colloids, such as the possibility of increased bleeding. An educational effort should be undertaken to disseminate guidelines regarding the appropriate indications for albumin, the therapeutic equivalence between artificial colloids and albumin, and evidence of artificial colloid safety.

Three categories of artificial colloids are available in Europe: dextrans, gelatins, and hydroxyethyl starches. Dextrans have some significant side effects concerning coagulation and renal function, which render their use less suitable in acute hemorrhagic shock. Allergic reactions to dextrans could be overcome by hapten inhibition. Gelatins do not interfere with the coagulation system. Accordingly, can be dosed at maximum effectiveness, which is an advantage in hemorrhagic conditions and especially in trauma. High-molecular-weight hydroxyethyl starches should be distinguished from those of medium molecular weight. The latter category is the most commonly used in European countries and is associated with good tolerance in terms of allegeric reactions and interference with coagulation. However, not all medium-molecular-weight hydroxyethyl starches are the same, especially when repeated infusions are considered. Acute renal failure following colloid administration has been reported with dextrans and hydroxyethyl starches but also with gelatins and 20% albumin. Risk factors and modes of administration have been identified as affecting these adverse events.

In this book, all the properties of artificial and natural colloids are reviewed. Different clinical settings that represent major indications for colloids are discussed extensively. Finally, we look to the future with the use of hemoglobin solutions and fluorocarbons.

Jean-Francois Baron and Johannes Treib

Contents

List of Contributors

AUDIBERT, GÉRARD, MD
Centre Hospitalier Universitaire
Service d'Anesthésie-Réanimation Chirurgical
29, avenue du Maréchal de Lattre de Tassigny
F-54035 Nancy Cédex

BALOGH, DORIS, Prof. Dr.
Leopold-Franzens-Universität Innsbruck
Univ.-Klinik für Anästhesie und Allgemeine Intensivmedizin
Anichstraße 35
A-6020 Innsbruck

BOLDT, JOACHIM, Prof. Dr.
Klinikum der Stadt Ludwigshafen
Abt. für Anästhesiologie und Intensivmedizin
Bremserstraße 79
D-67063 Ludwigshafen

CASAS, JUAN I., Dr.
Hospital de la Santa Cruz y San Pablo
Unidad Cuidados Intensivos-Cirurgia Cardiaca
Avda. Sant Antoni Maria Claret, 167
E-08025 Barcelona

EDWARDS, J.D., FRCP
University Hospital of South Manchester
Nell Lane
Manchester M20 2LR
United Kingdom

HALJAMÄE, HENGO, MD, PhD
Sahlgrenska University Hospital
Department of Anaesthesiology and Intensive Care
S-413 45 Göteborg

HIMPE, DIRK, Dr.
Middelheim General Hospital Antwerp
Division of Cardiac Anesthesia
Lindenreef 1
B-2020 Antwerp 2

LAXENAIRE, MARIE-CLAIRE, Prof. Dr.
Centre Hospitalier Universitaire
Service d'Anesthésie-Réanimation Chirurgical
29, avenue du Maréchal de Lattre de Tassigny
F-54035 Nancy Cédex

LITVAN, HÉCTOR, Dr.
Hospital de la Santa Cruz y San Pablo
Unidad Cuidados Intensivos-Cirurgia Cardiaca
Avda. Sant Antoni Maria Claret, 167
E-08025 Barcelona

SPAHN, DONAT R., Prof. Dr.
UniversitätsSpital Zürich
Institut für Anästhesiologie
Rämisstraße 100
CH-8091 Zürich

STOLL, MARTIN, Dr.
University of the Saarland
Department of Neurology
D-66421 Homburg

VILLAR-LANDEIRA, JUAN M., Dr.
Hospital de la Santa Cruz y San Pablo
Unidad Cuidados Intensivos-Cirurgia Cardiaca
Avda. Sant Antoni Maria Claret, 167
E-08025 Barcelona

Chapter 1

Albumin: To Use or Not to Use? Contemporary Alternatives?

1

H. Haljamäe

Introduction

Well balanced plasma volume support is essential in the clinical therapy of critically ill patients and patients undergoing elective or acute surgical procedures. The main objectives of the volume support are to maintain/achieve normovolaemia, haemodynamic stability, and adequate microvascular blood flow. An optimal fluid regimen should not include any obvious risk of excessive increases in tissue hydration, whereby microvascular blood flow may be jeopardized due to oedema induced compression of capillaries. The infusion of vast quantities of balanced salt solutions for plasma volume support may include such disadvantages due to the poor intravascular retention of a crystalloid [1]. When colloid containing solutions are infused, the presence of oncotically active macromolecules, which do not easily cross capillary membranes, will considerably reduce the total fluid volume requirements for adequate plasma volume support [1]. Therefore, plasma volume replacement with colloids is usually advantageous in many clinical situations [1, 2].

The dominating groups of commonly used artificial colloids for volume replacement are dextrans (Dex, 40,000–70,000 daltons), gelatins (Gel, succinylated, di-isocyanate urea-linked, or dialdehyde cross-linked; ~30,000–35,000 daltons), different hydroxyethyl starches (HES, 40,000–450,000 daltons), preparations including pentastarch (modified HES), and pentafractions of HES with more homogeneous molecular weight ranges [2]. The use of these artificial colloids in different clinical situations may be associated with advantages as well as disadvantages [2]. Albumin, being a natural colloid, has therefore by many clinicians been thought of as the ideal colloid for clinical use. During the last 5–10 years, however, routine use of albumin for volume replacement has been questioned [3–5]. The clinical indications for albumin seem rather controversial and aspects of cost efficiency and ethics are often included in the pro and con albumin discussions. In the present survey the physiological characteristics of albumin are summarised, risks associated with hypoalbuminaemia are discussed, and present indications for the use of albumin in different clinical situations are considered. Furthermore, characteristics of clinical importance of contemporary alternative colloids for volume replacement are summarised.

Albumin: The Natural Colloid

Physiological Characteristics of Albumin

Albumin, having a molecular mass of about 66,000–69,000 daltons, is the dominating plasma protein (about 45 g/l) (Table 1.1). It is synthesised by the liver and represents close to 50% of hepatic protein production [6]. Albumin synthesis is stimulated by the colloid osmotic pressure (COP) around the hepatocytes. Normally 130–200 mg/kg body weight is released daily from the liver and the total exchangeable albumin pool is 4–5 g/kg body weight of which 40% is intravascular and 60% extravascular (interstitial). The half-life of albumin is approximately 20 days. The equilibration time of exogenous albumin with the extravascular pool is in the range of 7–10 days.

Albumin is the major oncotically active plasma protein, contributing about 60%–80% of the plasma COP, which is in the range of 25–28 mm Hg [7]. About 18–20 mm Hg of plasma COP is caused by dissolved protein while 8–10 mm Hg is due to cations held in the plasma by the Donnan effect (the electronegative charges) of the proteins. Albumin is consequently of major importance in the regulation of transvascular fluid fluxes. Since albumin reversibly binds anions as well as cations, it is, in addition, a major transport protein for metals, free fatty acids, hormones, enzymes,

Table 1.1. Plasma proteins and physiological importance of albumin

Plasma proteins	(g/l)
– Albumin	(45)
– Globulins	(25)
– Fibrinogen	(3)
Total	(~70)
Adults	(65–80)
Children	(45–75)

Physiological importance
– Regulation of transvascular fluid flux
– Reversible binding of anions and cations
– Transport of FFA, hormones, enzymes, trace elements, drugs, etc.
– Detoxifying effects
– Scavenging of free radicals
– Inhibitory effect on platelet aggregation

drugs, etc. [8]. Furthermore, albumin has detoxifying effects, contributes to scavenging of free radicals, and exerts inhibitory effects on platelet aggregation (Table 1.1). It is thus obvious that albumin has rather unique features and that it plays an important role in the physiological homeostasis of the milieu interieur of the body [9].

Albumin Levels and Fluid Exchange in Critical Illness

Critical illness is usually associated with a reduction in the serum albumin level. This is partly due to reduced albumin synthesis since the production of acute phase reactants (such as globulins, fibrinogen, haptoglobin, etc.) is favoured as part of the stress mediated metabolic response occurring in the seriously ill individual. These phase reactants influence plasma COP which explains the observed poor correlation between plasma albumin levels and COP in critical illness [3].

A contributing factor to reduced serum albumin levels in the intensive care patient may be increased capillary permeability resulting in a net flux of albumin from the intra- to the extravascular space. Thereby, the fluid balance between the two different

fluid spaces will be disturbed and tissue oedema formation is favoured. It has been claimed that altered transcapillary protein flux
due to hypoalbuminaemia and/or increased capillary permeability
may critically enhance the risk of noncardiac pulmonary oedema
formation [10, 11]. However, experimental studies in primates
have demonstrated that although extreme reduction of plasma
COP, by 76%, will result in fluid retention, weight gain, peripheral
oedema, and ascites, no significant pulmonary oedema formation
will take place [12]. The lungs seem protected from oedema formation by a compensatory decrease in pulmonary interstitial COP
and a many-fold increase in lymph flow. In the above referred to
study, by Zarins et al. [12], however, isobaric capillary pressure
(Pc) conditions were at hand. A reduction of plasma COP will
also influence and reduce the critical Pc at which the rate of pulmonary oedema formation is increased [13]. It seems, however,
that the danger of pulmonary oedema due to low albumin levels
has been overestimated in clinical practice. Therefore, excessive
use of albumin with associated high costs may, in many clinical
situations, not be a physiologically justified routine.

Hypoalbuminaemia and Clinical Outcome

Clinically it was customary for quite a number of years to consider hypoalbuminemia to be associated with increased complication
rates, impaired wound healing, prolonged hospital stay, and increased mortality rates. Morissette et al. [14], in the mid-1970s,
reported dramatically increased mortality rates in patients with
lowered COP. The survival rates were 85% for patients with COP
≥18.5 mm Hg as compared to 0% for patients having COP
<10.5 mm Hg. However, more recent summaries of clinical out-
come data fail to verify significant correlations between high albumin levels and low incidence of complications or low mortality
rates [4]. Foley et al. [15], randomising critically ill patients either
to albumin supplementation to keep serum albumin >25 g/l or to
no supplementation, have reported that albumin supplementation
may rather increase mortality and morbidity rates. Their conclusion was that the costly use of exogenous albumin as treatment of

hypoalbuminaemia in the critically ill patient population did not appear to be justified, especially since there is growing concern over cost containment in health care systems. This is in agreement with other clinical studies [16, 17], on the basis of which Blackburn and Driscoll [5], in an editorial comment, suggested that it may be time to abandon routine albumin supplementation. Since hypoalbuminaemia is a normal phenomenon in the critically ill patient, albumin supplementation will only result in a transitory increase in the serum level but not really influence the clinical course [17]. In spite of such clinical data the serum albumin level has in recent years been included as a prognostic indicator in the Acute Physiology and Chronic Health Evaluation (APACHE III) illness severity scoring system [18].

Albumin in Shock Resuscitation

In shock and trauma situations some of the specific features of albumin, such as scavenging of free radicals [19] and anticoagulant properties, including inhibiting effects on platelet aggregation and enhancement of the inhibition of factor Xa caused by antithrombin III [20, 21], may be beneficial for moderation of the trauma induced activation of the coagulation cascade. In spite of these potentially beneficial effects, however, the use of albumin in clinical practice for intravascular volume expansion in shock and trauma patients has remained a matter of controversy [1, 2, 22–27].

There are several possible physiological explanations for potentially adverse effects of albumin in shock resuscitation. The pharmacokinetics of exogenously administered albumin is primarily determined by the distribution of albumin within the intra- and extravascular compartments. Since the intravascular pool of albumin is smaller (40%) than the extravascular pool (60%), the plasma volume supporting efficacy of albumin will be primarily determined by the dynamic equilibrium between these two pools. Due to the rather rapid exchange of exogenous albumin with the extravascular pool, the plasma volume expansion exerted by a 5% albumin solution is less pronounced than that seen, e.g. following infusion of dextran or HES [28]. The duration of the plasma volume support is therefore also of rather short duration, 1.5–4 h, and depends on how severely capillary permeability is affected. Trauma induced changes in capillary permeability will consequently result in increased transcapillary flux of albumin and reduce the plasma volume supporting capacity of albumin containing resuscitation fluids [1, 2]. At the same time the extravascular albumin content will increase, and "trapped" albumin in the interstitial tissue has been considered to increase the extravascular fluid content. In agreement with such a hypothesis Lucas et al. [23, 24] have reported detrimental effects of albumin on pulmonary function in trauma patients in response to the interstitial albumin trapping. Impairment of saline diuresis following albumin resuscitation was considered an important component for the detrimental effects of albumin on cardiopulmonary function [23, 25]. Lucas et al. [25] also observed that albumin treated patients had greater dependency on ventilatory support, averaging 8 days as compared to 3 days for patients not receiving albumin. On the basis of the harmful effects of albumin on fluid balance, and pulmonary and renal function, Lucas et al. [23] argued strongly against albumin supplementation for shock treatment. A negative inotropic effect of albumin on cardiac function has furthermore been suggested [26]. Such a cardiac effect could be partly related to binding of calcium to albumin whereby the level of ionised calcium is acutely reduced.

In experimental haemorrhagic shock, not including trauma, obvious detrimental effects of albumin resuscitation on organ function do not seem to be demonstrable [27]. Trauma induced activation of the cascade systems resulting in a systemic inflammatory response syndrome may therefore explain the clinical observations by Lucas et al. [23–25]. No advantage of albumin over artificial colloids in the resuscitation of critically ill shock and trauma patients in the clinical setting seems to be demonstrable [1, 2]. Use of albumin rather than 3.5% polygeline in critically ill patients has, e.g. not been found to influence clinical outcome or duration of stay in the intensive care unit [28], in spite of the relatively poor plasma volume supporting capacity of gelatin [1, 2, 29].

Although beneficial effects of albumin in the resuscitation of critically ill patients have been demonstrated [30, 31] the fact remains that hypoalbuminaemia may be regarded as a "normal" phenomen in the critically ill patient. The cost of routine administration of albumin on the basis of reduced plasma albumin levels may consequently not be justified especially since there is still a lack of conclusive data showing that such a therapy will significantly reduce morbidity or mortality [17, 32].

Albumin in Perioperative Volume Replacement

In spite of some physiological basis for potentially beneficial clinical effects of albumin for plasma volume substitution, the arguments against such a routine are becoming more and more dominating. Surgical injury will locally activate inflammatory cascades and increase capillary permeability. After major operative procedures there will be a shift of albumin from plasma into the interstitial fluid space with preferential binding in the skin and muscle surrounding the operative wound [17]. As part of the acute phase response evoked by the surgical trauma the production of acute phase reactants will be favoured at the expense of albumin synthesis. Therefore, perioperative albumin supplementation will only exert a transitory effect on the serum albumin concentration. In open heart surgery such an increase in albumin concentration and COP are demonstrable after albumin infusion but these changes do not seem to be associated with any significant clinical benefits [4]. The clinical value of such a transitory COP effect may consequently be questioned and, as pointed out by Alexander et al. [33] in 1989, albumin utilisation, also in a university hospital, may to a considerable extent (74%) be inappropriate. A more recent observational study by Yim et al. [34], characterising the prescribing of albumin in United States academic health centres, shows that albumin administration still is inappropriate in 62% of the cases. De Gaudio [35], in a recent review on the therapeutic use of albumin, states:

- Exogenous albumin is not an ideal colloid.
- The effects on plasma volume expansion are not entirely predictable, especially in pathological states accompanied by leaky capillary membranes.
- Albumin supplementation shows no benefit on many kinds of tissue oedema.

• The supplementation of albumin has no influence on outcome.

In specific clinical situations albumin supplementation may still be of value. Very low COP values and COP-WP (pulmonary capillary wedge pressure) differences ($\leqslant 3$ mm Hg) have been reported weakly to relate to survival, occurrence of adult respiratory distress syndrome, and formation of pulmonary oedema [36]. In many situations, however, artificial colloids may be as effective for plasma volume support and may even offer certain advantages over albumin [2]. In the postoperative period after abdominal surgery, including aortic surgery, it has even been suggested that albumin may be replaced by a 1.5 to two times higher volume of Ringer solution [37].

Consensus Statements for the Use of Albumin

There is an obvious need for institutions to define and implement guidelines that focus on the use of albumin for volume replacement in the clinical environment so that a cost-efficient use can be achieved. Consensus statements, based on assessment of albumin transfusion decision triggers in different clinical situations at different hospitals in various countries, have in recent years considerably influenced the discussions on the proper indications for albumin as plasma volume expander [33–40]. The scientific usefulness of such consensus conferences may be questioned but the consensus statements will probably diminish the abuse of albumin and improve medical practice. Consensus recommendations from 1992 for the use of albumin [41] include the following indications:

• Massive haemorrhage
• Plasmapheresis
• Massive hypoalbuminaemia
• Volume expansion in pregnancy

A more recent, systematic, literature-based consensus exercise, including 31 medical and allied health professionals in the USA [40], provides more complex clinical practice guidelines which may assist health care providers to develop local institutional policies for the appropriate and efficient use of albumin and albumin alternatives [40].

Contemporary Alternative Colloids

In many clinical situations artificial colloids may be used instead of albumin. In the choice of colloid important colloid characteristics such as the plasma volume expanding efficacy, haemorheologic effects, and possible influences on haemostatic competence have to be considered [2]. In Table 1.2 some colloid characteristics are summarised for different Dex and HES preparations as well as for

Table 1.2. Initial plasma volume supporting capacity, duration of the plasma volume expansion, haemorheologic effects, and influence on haemostatic function of some commonly used artificial plasma volume expanders. (Modified from [2])

	Initial plasma volume support	Duration of intravascular persistence	Haemorheo-logical effects	Haemostatic competence
Artificial colloid				
Dex 6%, MW 70,000	Good	Prolonged	Pronounced	Reduced
Dex 3%, W 60,000	Moderate	Prolonged	Pronounced	Reduced
Dex 10%, MW 40,000	Pronounced	Moderate	Pronounced	Reduced
HES 3%, MW 200,000	Moderate	Prolonged	Good	Reduced?
HES 6%, MW 200 000	Good	Prolonged	Good	Reduced?
HES 10%, MW 200,000	Good	Prolonged	Good	Reduced?
HES 6%, MW 450,000	Good	Prolonged	Good	Reduced
Gel 35 mg/ml	Poor	Limited	Limited	Unchanged?
Pentastarch/ fraction	Good	Prolonged	Good	Reduced?

Gel and pentastarch. Furthermore, the risk of colloid associated adverse reactions must be considered at the choice of artificial colloid.

Plasma Volume Supporting Capacity

The plasma volume expanding efficacy of a colloidal fluid is dependent on the size and concentration of the colloid-osmotically active molecules and their intravascular persistence. The COP of a plasma expander will influence its initial plasma volume expanding capacity. Intravenous infusion of colloids with a COP lower than or equal to that of plasma will result in a mainly isovolaemic initial plasma volume expansion. Colloids with a COP higher than that of plasma, by contrast, will have a greater initial plasma volume expanding capacity than the actual fluid volume infused. This is explained by colloid-osmotic mobilisation of fluid from extravascular sources into the intravascular compartment [1].

The more prolonged plasma volume supporting capacity of a colloid is determined by the numbers, sizes, and configurations of the molecules in the suspension and the breakdown and elimination characteristics for the substance [1]. The medium to high molecular Dex (60,000–70,000) and HES (200,000–450,000) preparations contain colloid molecules that do not easily leak across capillary membranes. Therefore, these colloids have moderate to good prolonged plasma volume supporting capacities lasting for hours. For the HES preparations the degree of molar substitution with hydroxyethyl groups will determine the speed of degradation by serum amylase and thereby influence the duration of the intravascular persistence. Therefore, the plasma volume support of HES preparations with a high degree of substitution is of longer duration than that of preparations with a lower degree of substitution. The degradation of pentastarch is more rapid than that of HES, i.e. the plasma volume expansion achieved with pentastarches is of shorter duration. Dex 40,000 and the different 3.5%–4% Gel preparations all contain relatively large proportions of low molecular weight components which rather rapidly will leak across semipermeable membranes. This is in agreement with the clinical observations by Lamke and Liljedahl

[29] when studying the plasma volume expansion achieved after infusion of 1 l of different plasma expanders to patients in the immediate postoperative period after moderate surgical procedures. They reported a remaining efficient plasma volume expansion of about 0.7–0.8 l for both 6% Dex 70,000 and HES (Volex) some 90 min after the infusion, while the plasma volume support of Gel (Haemaccel) was found to be only about 0.2 l, i.e. similar to that observed for physiological saline. Therefore, the authors concluded that Gel is not an efficient plasma expander when hypovolaemia is to be corrected rapidly. More recent clinical data have indicated a relatively adequate initial plasma volume expanding capacity of Gel (modified fluid gelatin – Gelofusine) for about 30 min [42]. The more prolonged intravascular retention of Gel, however, seems rather insignificant due to rapid redistribution and excretion. Østgaard and Onarheim [43] have recently experimentally studied the retention and distribution of polygeline (Haemaccel). They reported an intravascular retention as low as 23% 60 min after a 60-min infusion while 43% of the colloid had been excreted in the urine, and 33% had disappeared into other compartments.

In clinical practice the pros and cons of the pronounced differences in initial and more long-lasting plasma volume supporting efficacies that characterise the different available colloids must be considered when choosing colloid for specific therapeutic situations [2].

Haemorheologic Effects

The rheologic behaviour of blood is altered in many clinical situations and haemorheologic aspects should always be included when choosing colloid for plasma volume support (Table 1.2). The haemorheologic effectiveness of a colloid is determined by its haemodilutional capacity in combination with its inherent specific pharmacological effects on red cell aggregation, platelet function, plasma viscosity, and blood corpuscle-endothelial cell interactions [44, 45].

The reduction of the haematocrit level of the blood by haemodilution seems to be the most important determinant for the rheologic effects and thereby for enhancement of tissue perfusion and oxygenation [46, 47]. Vascular resistance is reduced by lowered whole blood viscosity which will enhance venous return and increase cardiac output [48]. In comparison to the dominating role played by haemodilution per se, changes in plasma viscosity seem of minor importance for alterations of tissue perfusion [49]. Both Dex and HES seem to increase plasma viscosity; however, the impact of plasma viscosity on the rheologic properties of whole blood has been shown to be completely offset by the concomitant reduction of haematocrit [50]. Therefore, no significant adverse effects of Dex or HES on tissue perfusion can be expected but rather enhancement of microvascular blood flow.

The plasma volume support obtained at the infusion of medium to high molecular Dex and HES/pentastarch preparations will effectively reduce haematocrit and thereby whole blood viscosity. This explains the advantageous haemorheologic effects of these types of artificial colloids (Table 1.2). However, low molecular weight (30,000–40,000) preparations of Dex and HES seem to induce even more pronounced beneficial haemorheologic effects [51].

Dex preparations are considered to induce somewhat more advantageous haemorheologic effects than HES preparations in spite of the similar plasma volume expanding capacities of both types of colloids (Table 1.2). The plasma volume expansion achieved at the infusion of Dex does not only result in haemodilution and reduced blood viscosity but also in disaggregation of erythrocytes, reduced platelet adhesiveness, and altered electronegativity of red blood cells and endothelial cell surfaces [52, 53]. Reduced red blood cell aggregation seems to constitute an important factor for the enhancement of blood flow, especially in the low pressure venous system. A possible more beneficial role of the pentafractions of HES than of regular HES in the inhibition of endothelial cell activation and neutrophil adhesion has been suggested [54]. Such an effect of HES may be related to a dose dependent inhibition of stimulated von Willebrand factor (vWF) release [55].

On the basis of presently available documentation the following order of haemorheologic effectiveness of artificial colloids is suggested [2]: dextran > pentastarch > hydroxyethyl starch > gelatin.

Therefore, in clinical situations, where rapid enhancement of microvascular blood flow is crucial for restitution of adequate tissue perfusion, Dex seems a better choice than HES or Gel. In spite of pronounced initial effects of low molecular (40,000) Dex on blood fluidity and thereby on tissue perfusion it seems that Dex 70,000 may be more favourable in many clinical situations, due to its better intravascular persistence and thereby more long-lasting haemorheologic effects.

Influences on Haemostatic Competence

Plasma volume expansion with artificial colloids will, in a colloid associated fashion, affect the haemostatic competence of the body [56]. The effects of a colloid on haemostasis are partly due to haemodilution resulting in decreased concentrations of coagulation factors and partly to colloid specific effects on the clotting of blood. As indicated in Table 1.2, the haemostatic competence is significantly reduced by Dex and high molecular weight (450,000) HES, while conclusive documentation of the clinical effects of medium molecular weight HES, pentastarch, and Gel on haemostasis has not been presented.

Dex is not an anticoagulant per se but it exerts antithrombotic effects by inducing haemodilution, enhancing microvascular blood flow, and modulating the haemostatic system. Combined effects of Dex on the concentration of coagulation factors, red blood cell aggregation, platelet activity, plasma levels of factor VIII, plasminogen activation, and plasma fibrinogen levels seem to all be factors contributing to the reduced haemostatic competence induced by Dex [45, 52]. The molecular structure and tensile behavior of fibrin is modulated by Dex so that clots formed in the presence of dextran are more fragile, which, together with the enhanced fibrinolytic activity, results in increased lysis of already formed clots. It has often been claimed that the use of Dex is limited in clinical practice due to its effects on haemostasis [57]. However, at intravenous dosages of Dex not exceeding 1.5 g/kg body weight per 24 h, the risk of haemorrhagic complications is insignificant in patients with undisturbed haemostasis prior to the infusion [58]. The combination of Dex with low molecular weight heparin (LMWH) seems to also be safe since no increased risk of bleeding has been reported when thromboprophylactic doses are administered and could even be beneficial [59].

HES solutions have been considered not to interfere with normal haemostasis [60]. Although conventional clotting parameters do not appear to be significantly affected, alterations seen as a von Willebrand-like syndrome and impairment of platelet function have been reported [61].

Infusion of larger volumes of high molecular weight (450,000) HES may, in particular, induce coagulopathy [62, 63]; while the use of medium molecular weight (200,000) HES or pentastarch seems to affect haemostasis to a lesser extent [64, 65]. The observed effect of rather small volumes of HES 200,000 on the activity of blood coagulation and fibrinolysis in healthy volunteers indicates that also medium molecular weight HES may influence haemostatic competence [65], and HES 200,000 associated increased blood loss has been reported [66].

Gel does not seem to influence haemostasis apart from a dose-dependent dilution of clotting factors [57, 66] although a risk haemorrhagic complications has been indicated by Watkins [67].

On the basis of the above considered documentation it may be concluded that the influence of artifical colloids on the haemostasic competence is roughly as follows [2]: dextran>HES 450,000 > HES 200,000 > pentastarch > gelatin.

Safe use of Dex and HES 450,000 requires that the maximal recommended dose of 1.5 g/kg body weight per 24 h is not exceeded. The risk of haemorrhagic complications at infusion of larger volumes of HES 200,000 or pentastarch may be somewhat smaller, but there seems to be a dose dependent influence on haemostasis, which should be considered when full haemostatic competence is needed.

Adverse Reactions to Artificial Colloids

Important aspects of colloid safety have recently been summarised by Ljungström [68]. General unspecific effects such as fluid overload, impairment of renal function, and dilution of plasma coagulation factors, as well as specific effects on certain plasma components

Table 1.3. Frequencies of severe allergic/anaphylactoid reactions reported for different colloids used for plasma volume support and for plasma [45]

	Dextran	HSA	HES	Gelatin	Plasma
Severe allergic/ anaphylactoid reactions (%)	0.001[a]	0.003	0.006	0.038	High

[a] Prophylaxis with monovalent hapten.

and cellular elements have to be taken into account. Plasma volume support with colloids may, in addition to the influences on haemostatic competence and renal function, also include a risk of colloid induced severe allergic and anaphylactoid reactions (Table 1.3).

It is a well known fact that infusion of plasma is associated with a higher incidence of hypotensive allergic/anaphylactoid reactions than infusion of any artificial colloid. Therefore, plasma is due to safety aspects not an optimal colloid. Gelatin seems to be the artificial colloid associated with the highest incidence of adverse reactions (Table 1.3). Lorenz et al. [69] have recently reported a very high incidence of histamine release and clinically relevant or even life-threatening cardiorespiratory disturbances when Haemaccel was infused during anaesthesia induction. Fatal reactions to Haemaccel have repeatedly been reported [70–72]. Therefore, Watkins [73] recently commented on the use of gelatins as follows: "Far from being inert substances, gelatins can readily initiate a life-threatening anaphylactoid response. Their formulations carry the risk of haemorrhagic complications too. Gelatins are not ideal as plasma expanders and should not be chosen routinely on the basis of cost alone." Urea-linked gelatin preparations seem to be associated with over twice the incidence of anaphylactoid reactions compared to the succinated form [57]. The fact remains, however, that the new modified preparations are also associated with an unacceptable incidence of allergic reactions [69]. This, in combination with the poor plasma volume supporting capacity and intravascular persistence of gelatin, makes gelatin preparations less suitable for resuscitation.

Previously, there was no evidence for the existence of preformed antibodies against HES in humans [74], and complement

activation was suggested to cause the rather uncommon allergic
reactions to HES [75]. Recently, however, high titres of HES specific antibodies have been detected in a patient reacting to HES
(200.000/0.5) in connection with aortic surgery [76]. HES resuscitation may in addition be associated with late, rather problematic
side effects seen as severe long-lasting pruritus appearing weeks
to months after the infusion [77, 78]. The itching seems related to
storage of HES in skin cells [78].

It is well known that dextran infusion may be associated with
hypersensitivity reactions [79, 80]. The mechanisms for the anaphylactoid reactions to dextran have been characterised in great
detail and the severe reactions have been shown to be related to
the presence of high titres of circulating dextran reactive antibodies of IgG class [81]. However, it is possible by preinjection of
dextran 1 to apply the hapten inhibition principle to clinical practice for prevention of dextran associated reactions [82, 83]. The
combination of any antidextran antibodies present in the recipient
with the low molecular weight (1000 dalton) dextran will result in
the formation of complexes too small to be reactive. The efficacy
and safety of this approach has been well documented [68, 84,
85]. Therefore, with hapten inhibition dextran seems to be the
safest plasma substitute in current clinical practice (Table 1.3).

Conclusions

Although albumin, from a physiological point of view, may be
considered an ideal natural colloid, its clinical use is not optimal
since inappropriate use of albumin still seems to be more common than appropriate use. A cost-conscious health care environment requires strict awareness among the different categories of
personnel involved in fluid therapy of the proper clinical indications for albumin. Therefore, there is a need for institutions to define and implement guidelines that focus on the use of albumin
for volume replacement in the clinical environment so that a cost-
efficient use can be achieved.

Artificial colloids constitute valuable alternatives to albumin in
many clinical situations. The use of any artificial colloid should be

based on proper knowledge of its specific colloid associated characteristics and the possible clinical implications of its effects on plasma volume, haemorheology, and haemostasis. Optimal clinical plasma volume management requires individualisation of the therapy since each individual colloid is associated with advantages and disadvantages in different clinical situations. Therefore, when choosing a colloid not only patient associated factors, such as underlying pathology, and cardiac, renal, and pulmonary functional status, but also plasma volume expander associated pharmacological and physiological effects have to be taken into account. Furthermore, the potential risk of colloid induced allergic/anaphylactoid reactions must be considered and whether effective prophylactic measures are available whereby the risk can be minimised.

■ **Acknowledgements.** Our own studies referred to in this survey were supported by grants from The Swedish Medical Research Council (project 05416), The Laerdal Foundation for Acute Medicine, The Göteborg Medical Society, and the LUA-project of the Medical Faculty, Göteborg University, and the Sahlgrenska University Hospital, Göteborg, Sweden.

References

1. Haljamäe H (1996) Crystalloids vs colloids. In: Risberg B (ed) Trauma care – an update. PR-Offset AB, Mölndal, Sweden, pp 129–41
2. Haljamäe H, Dahlqvist M, Walentin F (1997) Artificial colloids in clinical practice: pros and cons. Baillière's Clin Anaesthesiol 11:49–79
3. Grootendorst AF, van Wilgenburg AGM, de Laat PHJM, van der Hoven B (1988) Albumin abuse in intensive care medicine. Intensive Care Med 14:554–447
4. Erstad BL, Gales BJ, Rappaport WD (1991) The use of albumin in clinical practice. Arch Intern Med 151:901–911
5. Blackburn GL, Driscoll DF (1992) Time to abandon routine albumin supplementation. Editorial. Crit Care Med 20:157–158
6. Rothschild MA, Oratz M, Schreiber SS (1972) Albumin synthesis. N Engl J Med 286:748–756
7. Lewis RT (1980) Albumin: role and discriminative use in surgery. Can J Surg 23:322–328

8. Tullis JL (1977) Albumin. I. Background and use. JAMA 237:355–360
9. Emerson Jr TE (1989) Unique features of albumin: a brief review. Crit Care Med 17:690–694
10. Allen SJ, Drake RE, Williams JP, Laine GA, Gabel JC (1987) Recent advances in pulmonary edema. Crit Care Med 15:963–970
11. Oppenheimer L (1990) Lung fluid movement and its relevance to the management of patients with increased lung water. Clin Intens Care 1:103–110
12. Zarins CK, Rice CL, Peters RM, Virgilio RW (1978) Lymph and pulmonary responses to isobaric reduction in plasma oncotic pressure in baboons. Circul Res 43:925–930
13. Oppenheimer L (1990) Lung fluid movement and its relevance to the management of patients with increased lung water. Clin Intens Care 1:103–110
14. Morissette M, Weil MH, Shubin H (1975) Reduction in colloid osmotic pressure associated with fatal progression of cardiopulmonary failure. Crit Care Med 3:115–117
15. Foley EF, Borlase BC, Dzik WH, Bistrian BR, Bendotti PN (1990) Albumin supplementation in the critically ill. A prospective, randomized trial. Arch Surg 125:739–742
16. Wojtysiak SL, Brown RO, Robertson D, Powers DA, Kudsk KA (1992) Effect of hypoalbuminemia and parenteral nutrition on free water excretion and electrolyte-free water resorption. Crit Care Med 20:164–169
17. Marik PE (1993) The treatment of hypoalbuminemia in the critically ill patient. Heart Lung 22:166–170
18. Knaus WA, Wagner DP, Draper EA, et al. (1991) The APACHE III prognostic system. Risk prediction of hospital mortality for critically ill hospitalized adults. Chest 100:1619–1636
19. Holt M, Ryall M, Campell A (1984) Albumin inhibits human polymorphonuclear leucocyte luminol dependent chemilumminescence: evidence for oxygen scavenging. Br J Exp Pathol 65:231–241
20. Jørgensen KA, Stoffersen E (1979) Heparin like activity of albumin. Thromb Res 16:573–578
21. Jørgensen KA, Stoffersen E (1980) On the inhibitory effect of albumin on platelet aggregation. Thromb Res 17:13–18
22. Lucas CE, Ledgerwood AM, Mammen EF (1982) Altered coagulation protein content after albumin resuscitation. Ann Surg 196:198–202
23. Lucas CE, Ledgerwood AM, Higgins RF (1979) Impaired salt and water excretion after albumin resuscitation for hypovolemic shock. Surgery 86:544–549
24. Lucas CE, Ledgerwood AM, Higgins RF, Weaver DW (1980) Impaired pulmonary function after albumin resuscitation from shock. J Trauma 20:446–451
25. Lucas CE, Weaver D, Higgins RF, Ledgerwood AM, Johnson SD, Bouwman DL (1978) Effects of albumin versus non-albumin resuscitation on plamsa volume and renal excretory function. J Trauma 18:564–570

26. Dahn MS, Lucas CE, Ledgerwood AM, Higgins RF (1979) Negative inotropic effect of albumin resuscitation for shock. Surgery 86:235–241
27. Layon AJ, Gallagher TJ (1990) Five percent human albumin in lactated Ringer's solution for resuscitation from hemorrhagic shock: Efficacy and cardiopulmonary consequences. Crit Care Med 18:410–413
28. Stockwell MA, Riley B (1992) Colloid solutions in the critically ill. A randomised comparison of albumin and polygeline. I. Outcome and duration of stay in the intensive care unit. Anaesthesia 47:3–6
29. Lamke L-O, Liljedahl S-O (1976) Plasma volume changes after infusion of various plasma expanders. Resuscitation 5:93–102
30. Shoemaker WC, Schluchter M, Hopkins JA, Appel PL, Schwartz S, Chang PC (1981) Comparison of the relative effectiveness of colloids and crystalloids in emergency resuscitation. Am J Surg 142:73–81
31. Rackow EC, Falk JL, Fein A, et al. (1983) Fluid resuscitation in circulatory shock: a comparison of the cardiorespiratory effects of albumin, hetastarch, and saline solutions in patients with hypovolemia and septic shock. Crit Care Med 11:839–850
32. Golub R, Sorrento Jr JJ, Cantu Jr R, Nierman DM, Moideen A, Stein HD (1994) Efficacy of albumin supplementation in surgical intensive care unit: A prospective, randomized study. Crit Care Med 22:613–619
33. Alexander MR, Stumpf JL, Nostrant TT, Khanderia U, Eckhauser FE, Colvin CL (1989) Albumin utilization in a university hospital. Ann Pharmacother 23:214–217
34. Yim JM, Vermeulen LC, Erstad BL, Matuszewski KA, Burnett DA, Vlasses PH (1995) Albumin and nonprotein colloid solution use in US academic health centers. Arch Intern Med 155:2450–2455
35. De Gaudio AR (1995) Therapeutic use of albumin. Int J Artif Organs 18:216–224
36. Shippy CR, Shoemaker WC (1983) Hemodynamic and colloid osmotic pressure alterations in the surgical patient. Crit Care Med 11:191–195
37. Blanloeil Y, Leteurnier Y, Francois T (1996). Indications and role of albumin for vascular loading during postoperative intensive care. Ann Fr Anesth Reanim 15:497–506
38. Subcommittee of the Victorian Drug Usage Advisory Committee (1992) Human albumin solutions: consensus statements for use in selected clinical situations. Med J Aust 157:340–343
39. Nicholls MD, Whyte G (1993) Red cell, plasma and albumin transfusion decision triggers. Anaesth Intens Care 21:156–162
40. Vermeulen LC, Ratko TA, Erstad BL, Brecher ME, Matuszewski MS (1995) A paradigm for consensus. The university hospital consortium guidelines for the use of albumin, nonprotein colloid, and crystalloid solutions. Arch Intern Med 155:373–379
41. Durand-Zaleski I, Bonnet F, Rochant H, Bierling P, Lemaire F (1992) Usefulness of consensus conferences: the case of albumin. Lancet 340:1388–1390

42. Beards SC, Watt T, Edwards JD, Nightingale P, Farragher EB (1994) Comparison of the hemodynamic and oxygen transport responsen to modified fluid gelatin and hetastarch in critically ill patients: A prospective, randomized trial. Crit Care Med 22:600–605

43. Østgaard G, Onarheim H (1996) Retention and distribution of polygeline (Haemaccel) in the rat. Acta Anaesthesiol Scand 40:96–101

44. Haljamäe H (1985) Pathophysiology of shock-induced disturbances in tissue homeostasis. Acta Anaesthesiol Scand 29, Suppl. 82:38–44

45. Arfors K-E, Buckley PB (1989) Role of artificial colloids in rational fluid therapy. In: Tuma RF, White JV, Messmer K (eds). The role of hemodilution in optimal patient care. München. Zuckswerdt, pp 100–123

46. Brückner UB, Messmer K (1991) Organ perfusion and tissue oxygenation after moderate isovolemic hemodilution with HES 200/0.62 and dextran-70. Anaesthetist 40:434–440

47. Le Veen HH, Ip M, Ahmed N, Mascardo T, Guinto RB, Falk G, D'Ovidio N (1980) Lowering blood viscosity to overcome vascular resistance. Surg Gynecol Obstet 150:139–149

48. Kouraklis G, Sechas M, Skalkeas G (1989) Effects of hemodilution on peripheral circulation. Vasc Surg 23:20–26

49. Brückner UB, Messmer K (1990) Blood rheology and systemic oxygen transport. Biorheology 27:903–912

50. Krieter H, Brückner UB, Kefalianakis F, Messmer K (1995) Does colloid-induced hyperviscosity in haemodilution jeopardize perfusion and oxygenation in vital organs? Acta Aneasthesiol Scand 39:236–244

51. Goto Y, Sakakura S, Hatta M, Sugiura Y, Kato T (1985) Hemorheologic effects of colloidal plasma substitutes infusion. A comparative study. Acta Anaesthesiol Scand 29:217–223

52. Bergqvist D, Bergentz S-E (1983) The role of dextran in severe ischemic extremity disease and arterial reconstructive surgery. VASA 12:213–218

53. Baldwin AL, Wu NZ, Stein DL (1991) Endothelial surface charge of interstitial mucosal capillaries and its modulation by dextran. Microvasc Res 42:160–178

54. Nolte D, Illner A, Menger MD, Messmer K (1992) Reduction of post-ischemic leukocyte-endothelium interaction by dextran 70 but not hydroxyethylstarch 200/0.62. Int J Microcirc: Clin Exp 11:203–226

55. Collis RE, Collins PW, Gutteridge CN et al. (1994) The effect of hydroxyethyl starch and other plasma volume substitutes on endothelial cell activation an in vitro study. Intensive Care Med 20:37–41

56. Strauss RG (1988) Volume replacement and coagulation: A comparative review. J Cardiothorac Anesth 2, Suppl. 1:24–32

57. Nearman HS, Herman ML (1991) Toxic effects of colloids in the intensive care unit. Crit Care Clin 7:713–723

58. Bergman A, Andreen M, Blombäck M (1990) Plamsa substitution with 3% dextran-60 in orthopaedic surgery: influence on plasma colloid osmotic pressure, coagulation parameters, immunoglobulins and other plasma constituents. Acta Anaesthesiol Scand 34:21–29

59. Matthiasson SE, Lindblad B, Mätzsch T, Molin J, Qvarfordt P, Bergqvist D (1994) Study of the interaction of dextran and enoxaparin on haemostasis in humans. Thromb Haemost 72:722–727

60. Claes Y, Hemelrijck JV, Van Gerven M, et al. (1992) Influence of hydroxyethyl starch on coagulation in patients during the perioperative period. Anesth Analg 75:24–30

61. Boldt J, Knothe C, Zickmann B, Andres P, Dapper F, Hempelmann G (1993) Influence of different intravascular volume therapies on platelet function in patients undergoing cardiopulmonary bypass. Anesth Analg 76:1185–1190

62. Strauss RG, Stump DC, Henriksen RA (1985) Hydroxyethyl starch accentuates von Willebrand's disease. Transfusion 25:235–237

63. Sanfelippo MJ, Suberviola PD, Geimer NF (1987) Development of a von Willebrand-like syndrome after prolonged use of hydroxyethyl starch. Am J Clin Pathol 88:653–655

64. Strauss RG, Stansfield C, Henriksen RA, Villhauer PJ (1988) Pentastarch may cause fewer effects on coagulation than hetastarch. Transfusion 28:257–260

65. Kapiotis S, Quehenberger P, Eichler H-G et al. (1994) Effect of hydroxyethyl starch on the activity of blood coagulation and fibrinolysis in healthy volunteers: Comparison with albumin. Crit Care Med 22:606–612

66. Mortelmans YJ, Vermaut G, Verbruggen AM, et al. (1995) Effects of 6% hydroxyethyl starch and 3% modified fluid gelatin on intravascular volume and coagulation during intraoperative hemodilution. Anesth Analg 81:1235–1242

67. Watkins J (1994) Reactions to gelatin plasma expanders. Letter to the editor. Lancet 344:328–329

68. Ljungström K-G (1997) Colloid safety: fact and fiction. Baillière's Clin Anaesthesiol 11:163–177

69. Lorenz W, Duda D, Dick W, et al. (1994) Incidence and clinical importance of perioperative histamine release: randomized study of volume loading and antihistamines after induction of anaesthesia. Lancet 343:933–940

70. Watkins J (1991) Allergic and pseudoallergic reactions to colloid plasma substitutes. Which colloid? Care Crit Ill 7:213–217

71. Lorenz W, Doenicke A, Messmer K, et al. (1976) Histamin release in human subjects by modified gelatin (haemaccel) and dextran: An explanation for anaphylactoid reactions observed under clinical conditions? Br J Anaesth 48:151–165

72. Freeman MK (1979) Fatal reaction to haemaccel. Anaesthesia 34:341–343

73. Watkins J (1994) Reactions to gelatin plasma expanders. Letter to the editor. Lancet 344:328–329

74. Kraft D, Sirtl C, Laubenthal H, et al. (1992) No evidence for the existance of preformed antibodies against hydroxyethyl starch in man. Eur Surg Res 24:138–142

75. Porter SS, Goldberg RJ (1986) Intraoperative allergic reactions to hydroxyethyl starch: a report of two cases. Can Anaesth Soc J 33:394–398
76. Kreimeier U, Christ F, Kraft D, et al. (1995) Anaphylaxis due to hydroxyethyl-starch-reactive antibodies. Lancet 346:49–50
77. Parker NE, Porter JB, Williams HJM, Leftley N (1982) Pruritus after administration of hetastarch. Br Med J 284:385–386
78. Jurecka W, Szépfalusi Z, Parth E, et al. (1993) Hydroxyethylstarch deposits in human skin – a model for pruritus? Arch Dermatol Res 285:13–19
79. Richter AW, Hedin HI (1982) Dextran hypersensitivity. Immunol Today 3:132–138
80. Laxenaire MC, Charpentier C, Feldman L, et al. (1994) Anaphylactoid reactions to colloid plasma substitutes: Frequency, risk factors and mechansisms. Ann Fr Anesth Réanim 13:301–310
81. Kraft D, Hedin H, Richter W, Scheiner O, Rumpold H, Devey M (1982) Immunoglobulin class and subclass distribution of dextran-reactive antibodies in human reactors and non-reactors to clinical dextran. Allergy 37:481–489
82. Hedin H, Richter W (1982) Pathomechanisms of dextran-induced anaphylactoid/anaphylactic reactions in man. Int Archs Allergy Appl Immun 68:122–126
83. Ljungström K-G, Renck H, Hedin H, Richter W, Wiholm B-E (1988) Hapten inhibition and dextran anaphylaxis. Anaesthesia 43:729–732
84. Ljungström KG, Willman B, Hedin H (1993) Hapten inhibition of dextran anaphylaxis. Nine years of post-marketing surveillance of dextran 1. Ann Fr Réanim 12:219–222
85. Ljungström K-G (1993) Safety of dextran in relation to other colloids – ten years experience with hapten inhibition. Infusionsther Transfusionsmed 20:206–210

CHAPTER 2

Use of Gelatins as Volume Expanders in Shock and Trauma

2

J.D. EDWARDS

Introduction

The most important function of the circulation is the transport of oxygen to the respiring tissues. Oxygen (O_2) is the most vital of all the substrates carried by the circulation yet compared to the rate of utilisation it has the lowest stores and its consumption is also uniquely flow rather than consumption dependent. Lack of O_2 does not only disrupt the function of the vital organs it may damage or completely destroy them. Therefore, the use of volume replacement theory in shock has to be considered in this context. The relationship between the delivery of oxygen (DO_2) and oxygen consumption (VO_2) is known as the oxygen transport (O_2T) system. This is primarily considered in quantitative terms; normal values are summarised in Fig. 2.1.

Note that at rest the normal DO_2 is such that 25% of available O_2 is consumed giving an oxygen extraction ratio (OER) of 25%

NORMAL OXYGEN TRANSPORT PATTERNS

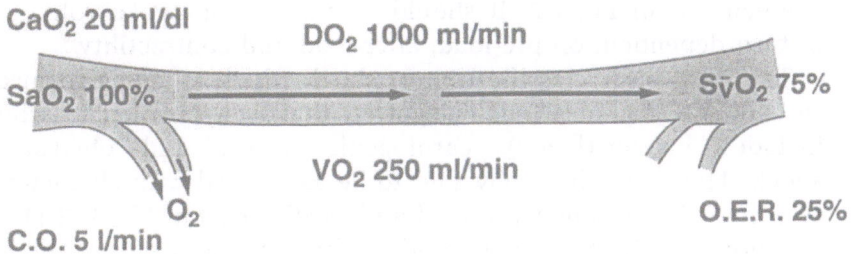

CaO_2 20 ml/dl DO_2 1000 ml/min

SaO_2 100% $S\bar{v}O_2$ 75%

VO_2 250 ml/min

O_2

O.E.R. 25%

C.O. 5 l/min

Fig. 2.1.

DETERMINANTS OF DO$_2$

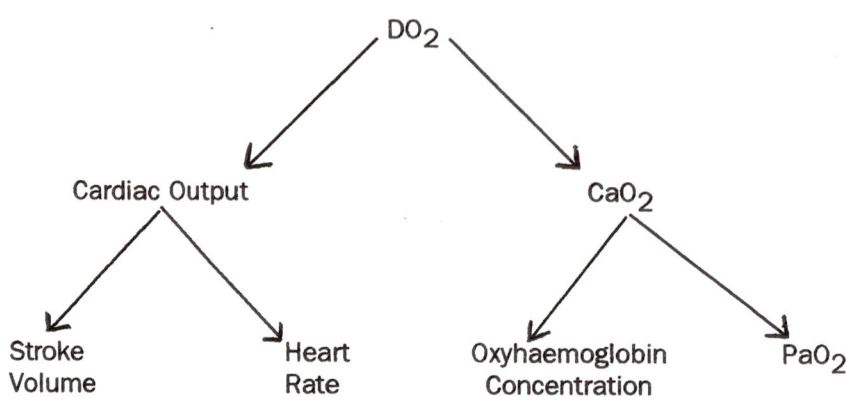

Fig. 2.2. Determinants of DO$_2$

Table 2.1. Classic haemodynamic classification of shock

Diagnostic category	PAOP	CO
Hypovolaemic	⇊	⇊
Septic	⇊	⇑
Cardiogenic	⇑	⇊
Obstructive	⇔	⇊

PAOP, pulmonary artery occlusion pressure; CO, cardiac output.

and a mixed venous oxyhaemoglobin saturation (S$_V$O$_2$) of 75%. In clinical practice, cardiac output (CO) is divided by body surface to derive cardiac index (CI) in l/min/m^2. A normal value of DO$_2$ when indexed is 550–600 l/min/m^2. The determinants of DO$_2$ are summarised in Fig. 2.2. It should be noted that stroke volume is in turn dependent on pre-load, after-load and contractility.

The most basic classification of shock which is taught to medical students includes four categories; that is hypovolemic (which includes haemorrhagic), cardiogenic, septic and obstructive shock. These are classically said to be associated with characteristic levels of ventricular pre-load and cardiac output (Table 2.1).

Unfortunately this simple model, while of use as a basis for initial understanding of the management of shock, does not apply to the majority of the critically ill patients who require intensive care management. For instance some patients with cardiogenic shock may have a critically low pulmonary artery occlusion pressure (PAOP), as shown by Edwards [1], and some patients with septic shock due to peritonitis may have levels of cardiac output which are as low as those seen in cardiogenic shock even after plasma volume expansion, as shown in the study by Vincent [2]. Similarly patients with blunt thoracic trauma and other injuries may suffer myocardial contusion and present with levels of oxygen delivery approaching those seen in cardiogenic shock following acute myocardial infarction [3]. Central to the current discussion is that after securing the airway and correcting hypoxaemia correction of relative or absolute hypovolaemia is the most important initial step in the management of all patients on the ICU.

The importance of fluid replacement therapy after trauma was highlighted by Cournand [4] in a study of unresuscitated trauma victims which demonstrated critically low levels of DO_2 and mixed S_VO_2 associated with low circulating plasma and blood volume and cardiac pre-load. This study highlighted the need for volume expansion in trauma victims, and coming as it did towards the end of World War II gave impetus to the development of artificial colloids. It also effectively ended the previous controversies concerning the cause of shock following trauma. We will not discuss aspects of blood transfusion although this is an equally important issue. However, use of colloid therapy has important effects on haematocrit and haemoglobin levels which may be of relevance to blood transfusion requirements as discussed below.

Principles of Volume Replacement

These have been comprehensively reviewed [5] recently and therefore only a bare outline will be given here. A reduced circulating blood volume, as a result of internal or external losses or relative hypovolaemia as a result of profound vasodilatation in septic or anaphylactic shock, impairs venous return to the heart and leads to reduced left ventricular pre-load. This is monitored at the bedside by measurement of PAOP but in actual fact is the left ventri-

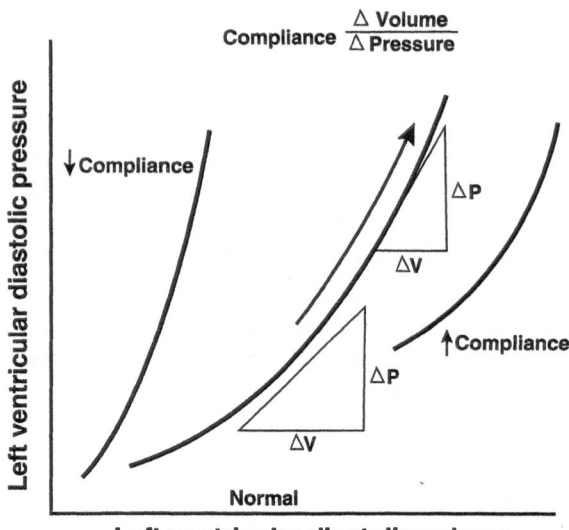

Fig. 2.3.

cular end diastolic volume. The relationship between pressure and volume is determined by the compliance of the left ventricle (Fig. 2.3).

For this reason no particular level of PAOP should be aimed for but volume therapy should be titrated by repeated measurements of PAOP, CO and calculations of stroke volume and left ventricular stroke work index (LVSWI) to construct a Frank-Starling or Sarnoff ventricular function curve respectively. Of course invasive monitoring is not required in the majority of cases initially. For instance patients with major trauma, cutaneous burns, acute gastroenteritis or peritonitis should receive fluid therapy, at least initially on clinical grounds alone. However, even here some refinements based on standard vital signs can be applied based on calculation of shock index [6]. This aspect is discussed in more detail below. However, if volume expansion guided by clinical signs fails then patients are referred for ICU therapy and it is under these circumstances that invasive monitoring with systemic and pulmonary arterial catheters is required, as clinical assessment of cardiac output, systemic vascular resistance and volume status are notoriously unreliable in severe circulatory shock.

Volume Replacement in Specific Clinical Situations

Trauma

Early theories on the aetiology of post-traumatic shock were reviewed by Cannon [7]. At that time, hypovolaemia was thought to be a contributory factor in only isolated cases. Popular theories included that of acarbia (shock secondary to hyperventilation), exhaustion of the vasomotor control centre, toxic myocardial depression and capillary stagnation. The latter being given particular attention by Cannon. Even though he underestimated the role of hypovolaemia, in a subsequent article he advocated use of up to 1 l of sodium bicarbonate in some cases [8]. However, pioneering laboratory work by Blalock [9] and the later milestone clinical paper by Cournand [4] established that hypovolaemia, even in the absence of obvious haemorrhage, was the prime abnormality in post-traumatic shock. Cournand's work involved measurement of cardiac output, circulating blood and plasma volume and measurement of arterial pH, blood lactate and S_VO_2. He did not take the final step and calculate DO_2 or VO_2, but his paper provides the raw data from which these calculations can be made. These are summarised in Fig. 2.4.

Our group prospectively studied 19 patients with major trauma within 4 h of their injury after correction of hypovolaemia and

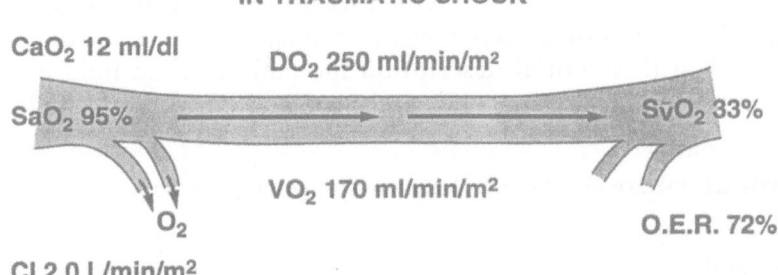

OXYGEN TRANSPORT PATTERNS
IN TRAUMATIC SHOCK

CaO_2 12 ml/dl DO_2 250 ml/min/m²

SaO_2 95% S_VO_2 33%

VO_2 170 ml/min/m²

O_2 O.E.R. 72%

CI 2.0 L/min/m²

Fig. 2.4. The effects of various fluids on cardiac index (CI) and blood volume (BV)

hypoxaemia. We found that VO_2 was normal or increased in all patients except those who were hypothermic [10]. In essence VO_2 is maintained at high normal levels in the face of very low levels of DO_2 by large increases in OER. That these are the characteristic oxygen transport findings in the immediate post injury phase have since been confirmed by several workers, including Moore [11] and Fleming [12].

Increasingly trauma resuscitation is based on Advanced Trauma Life Support (ATLS) guidelines [13]. These emphasise the importance of assessing the size of the injury as well as monitoring vital signs. The degree of haemorrhage in terms of the amount of circulating blood volume lost is assessed by basic clinical signs (Table 2.2).

The priorities of resuscitation are *airways, breathing, circulation, disability* and *exposure*. Colloid solutions appear to be unpopular in the United States as gelatin solutions are currently unavailable and the choice is therefore limited to albumin, starch or dextran preparations which all have severe limitations. Initially two long bore (16 or 14G) cannulas are placed and 2 l of Ringer's lactate are administered rapidly. With suitable experience a surgeon can rapidly perform a cut-down on the superficial proximal part of the long saphenous vein. Catheters used for central venous pressure monitoring have inadequate flow rates for fluid administration after trauma but a pulmonary artery introducer sheath (7.5FG) can be placed in the internal or external jugular or femoral vein if the necessary surgical expertise for cut-down is not readily available. The subclavian vein is best avoided.

There has been some controversy concerning the possible role of fluid administration in the aetiology of acute respiratory distress syndrome (ARDS) [14, 15] which led to veiled recommendation of fluid limitation or diuretics in the management of such cases [16]. Indeed in their initial description the authors cited fluid overload as an aetiological factor [17], and Pepe and co-workers cited trans-

Table 2.2. Intravenous fluid replacement in hemorrhagic shock

Class I hemorrhage	750 ml (15%)
Class II hemorrhage	800–1500 ml (15%–30%)
Class III hemorrhage	1500–2000 ml (30%–40%)
Class IV hemorrhage	2000 ml (48%)

fusions as a risk factor [18]. However, in that study, the initial PaO_2/FIO_2 ratio taken immediately after intubation and before significant transfusion correlated inversely with the eventual development of ARDS suggesting that pulmonary damage was present before fluid administration. Also Shoemaker and his co-workers have demonstrated that non-survivors of post-traumatic ARDS had higher blood volume deficits at all stages of the illness [19]. This suggests strongly that uncorrected hypovolaemia may contribute to the mortality in ARDS. It has long been recognised that patients with ARDS rarely die of hypoxaemia but usually with multi-system organ failure (MSOF) [20, 21], and there is evidence that this is related to inadequate levels of DO_2. Russel and co-workers, in a heterogeneous group of 29 patients, found that mean DO_2 was 718 ± 163 ml/min/m^2 in survivors compared to 491 ± 219 ml/min/m^2 in non-survivors [22]. Our group presented similar findings in 100 patients [23] with DO_2 being consistently higher and OER consistently lower at all recorded times (Table 2.3).

Table 2.3.

	S Mean±SD		NS Mean±SD		p Value
Initial					
DO_2 (ml/min/m^2)	745	234	660	276	<0.05
VO_2 (ml/min/m^2)	147	33	145	47	ns
OER%	19.9	5	23.9	7.4	<0.01
Highest					
DO_2 (ml/min/m^2)	1131	252	1022	272	<0.05
VO_2 (ml/min/m^2)	198	34	193	42	ns
OER%	20.6	2.6	19.6	4.3	<0.05
Lowest					
DO_2(ml/min/m^2)	563	112	502	135	0.05
VO_2 (ml/min/m^2)	135	36	129	31	ns
OER%	24.6	7	27.0	7.6	ns
Highest ABL (mmol/l)	2.6	1.8	3.1	2.6	ns

S, survivors; NS, non-survivors; SD, standard deviation; DO, oxygen delivery; VO, oxygen consumption; OER, oxygen extraction ratio; ABL, arterial blood lactate; ns, not significant.

Perhaps more significantly when we examined the relationship between ARDS, MSOF and survival in patients with blunt thoracic trauma there was a significant difference in the initial value of DO_2 and OER between the group with MSOF and poor survival compared to those without MSOF [23]. There were no differences in Total Injury Severity Score (ISS) and Abbreviated Injury Score (AIS) for the chest between the two groups (Table 2.4).

The O_2T variables given in Table 2.4 were derived after controlled volume expansion on the ICU with modified fluid gelatin (MFG) and packed red blood cells – guided by repeated measurements of PAOP, haemoglobin concentration and calculations of LVSWI. It was our impression that many of these patients were under-transfused before ICU admission; we therefore prospectively studied a further group of multiple trauma victims and recorded haemodynamic and O_2T data immediately on ICU admission [24]. We found that under-transfusion was common with PAOP values below 10 mm Hg in the majority of cases with subsequent increases in DO_2 after further volume and red blood cell transfusion.

Unfortunately in 17 cases fluid therapy was limited because central venous pressure (CVP) was measured and found to be high. In this study we found no correlation between CVP and PAOP

Table 2.4. Pattern of injury and organ failure after chest injuries

	Group 1 $(n = 9)$	Group 2 $(n = 15)$	p^*
Age (years)	46(25)	35(17)	ns
Chest AIS	4(0.5)	4(0.6)	ns
Total Injury Severity Score	32(13)	26(8)	ns
ARDS	9	8	<0.05
ARF	3	0	<0.05
Number of deaths	7	2	<0,05
Patients with abdominal injuries	5	7	ns
Patients with craniospinal injuries	5	8	ns
Patients with limb injuries	9	10	ns

Values are mean (sd); chest AIS, Abbreviated Injury Scale score for the chest; ARDS, acute respiratory distress syndrome; ARF, acute respiratory failure; ns, not significant; $^*\chi^2$ test.

and we recommend that fluid management by CVP after major trauma is not carried out.

Major Burns with Acute Respiratory Distress Syndrome

Rather surprisingly there is little published data on the haemodynamic and O_2T variables in the early phases following thermal cutaneous burns in humans and there has been controversy concerning the role of fluid therapy in the aetiology of ALI following burns with or without smoke inhalation injury. Dries and Waxman [25] showed that monitoring of so-called vital signs did not provide a reliable estimate of pre-load, CO or DO_2 in burns patients.

We conducted a retrospective study of cardiorespiratory patterns in survivors and non-survivors of patients with major burns with respiratory failure [26]. Prior to ICU admission all patients had ostensibly been resuscitated according to a standard burns formula. When initial measurements of PAOP and DO_2 were compared between survivors and non-survivors they were significantly higher in survivors with in the first 36 h. Survivors also had a higher net positive fluid balance and it was obvious that fluid requirements had been grossly underestimated in non-survivors despite there being no difference between the degree of pulmonary insufficiency as judged by the estimated alveolar to arterial oxygen tension difference [$P(A-a)O_2$] (Table 2.5). Once again in many patients fluid therapy had been withheld because CVP had been measured and found to be high.

Table 2.5. Early cardiorespiratory patterns in patients with major burns and respiratory failure

	S	±SEM	NS	±SEM
$P(A-a)O_2$ kPa	41.2	6.8	42.2	5.0
QS/QT (%)	23.4	3.4	28.5	3.8
DO_2 (ml/min/m^2)	782	55	864	79
VO_2 (ml/min/m^2)	140	18	146	14
OER (%)	17.7	2.1	29.4	11.7
PAOP (mm Hg)	13.0	3.0	8.0	1.5

O₂T Responses to Different Colloids

The variability in responses to different fluids was shown by Shoe-maker [27], who compared the relative effectiveness of whole blood, dextran 70 and 40, albumin and two crystalloid solutions on increasing CO and blood volume. In summary, 1 l of crystal-loid had minimal effect on either of these variables whereas col-loid, in particular dextran 40, produced large increases in both. A further study from the same group [28] compared newer available colloids – hydroxyethylated starch (HES) and salt-poor albumin and demonstrated even greater variability (Fig. 2.5).

In that study the authors demonstrated the poor predictive val-ue of changes in individual values of vital signs, central venous pressure (CVP) and even PAOP on CO and blood volume. In both these studies, blood volume was estimated using radioactive tech-niques which were not suitable for routine bedside management. It will be seen from Fig. 2.4 that of the colloids studied HES pro-

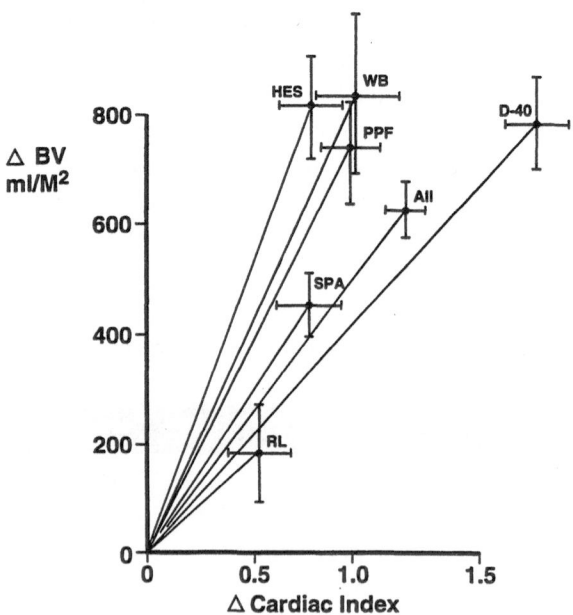

Fig. 2.5.

duced the largest increase in blood volume but the smallest increase in CO. In that study a significant fall in haematocrit (up to 10%) was seen in the group as a whole. In two related studies Haupt [29] and Gilbert [30] demonstrated a reduction in DO_2 in 20%–30% of critically ill septic patients in response to HES. In the first study, six of 20 patients showed reductions in DO_2 from 518±180 ml/min/m^2 to 475±160 ml/min/m^2 as the reduction in haematocrit outweighed the minimal increases in CO. The danger of this effect was highlighted in two other studies [31, 32] which showed that a significant proportion of critically ill surgical patients with apparently low left ventricular pre-load responded to volume expansion with a fall in CO.

In ten patients with clinical and haemodynamic features of circulatory shock our group studied the effects of rapid infusion of 0.5 l MFG [33]. The results are summarised in Table 2.6.

Once again a significant reduction in arterial oxygen content (CaO_2) due to haemodilution was noted but in this case the falls were minimal and increases in CO were more than sufficient to compensate. Therefore, there were significant increases in DO_2. Note that there were no significant falls in heart rate despite in-

Table 2.6. Hemodynamic and oxygen transport variables after rapid infusion of 500 ml MFG (mean±SD)

Variable	Control	T15	T30
HR (beat/min)	88±17	83±15	87±21
MAP (mmHg)	67±26	73±25	84±22[a]
WP (mmHg	4±3	10±4[a]	12±3[a]
CI (L/min·m^2)	3.4±1.6	4.1±1.7[a]	4.6±1.9[a]
SI (ml/m^2)	36±14	45±14[a]	49±9[a]
LVSWI (g·m/m^2)	33±18	40±18	47±18[a]
RVSWI (g·m/m^2)	7±5	10±8	12±8[a]
SVRI (dyne·sec/cm^5·m^2)	1586±741	1315±538	1246±384
QSP/Qt (%)	28±11	25±11	25±11
Hgb (g/dl)	10.9±2.4	10.2±1.9	9.9±1.8[a]
CaO$_2$ (ml/dl)	14.9±3.1	13.9±2.4	13.5±2.4[a]
DO$_2$(ml/min·m^2)	455±219	525±234	578±244[a]
VO, (ml/min·m^2)	102±39	119±38	135±39[b]

[a] p<0.5 vs control; [b] p=0.089 vs control; SVRI = systemic vascular resistance index.

creases in cardiac index (CI) and stroke volume index (SVI). Also there was no correlation between CVP and PAOP either before or after volume expansion. We shall emphasise this point repeatedly.

Comparative Studies in Sepsis and ARDS

Rackow's group compared the effects of a new low molecular weight hydroxyethyl starch, pentastarch, to albumin in a group of septic patients [34]. Although the cardiac output responses were

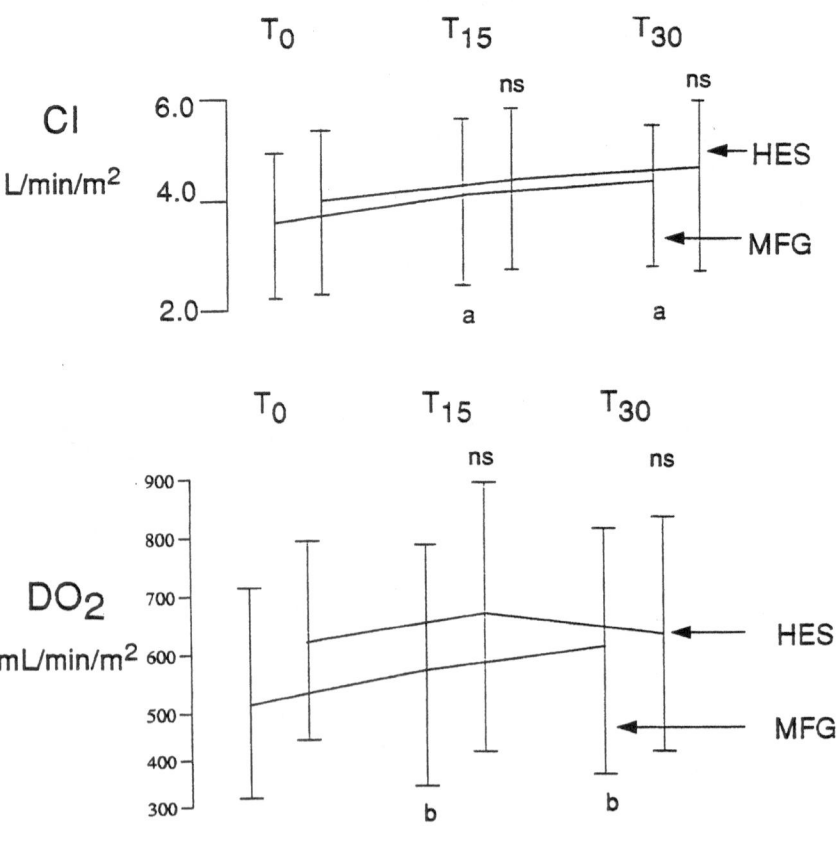

a = p <0.01, b = p <0.05, ns = non-significant compared to T_0

Fig. 2.6

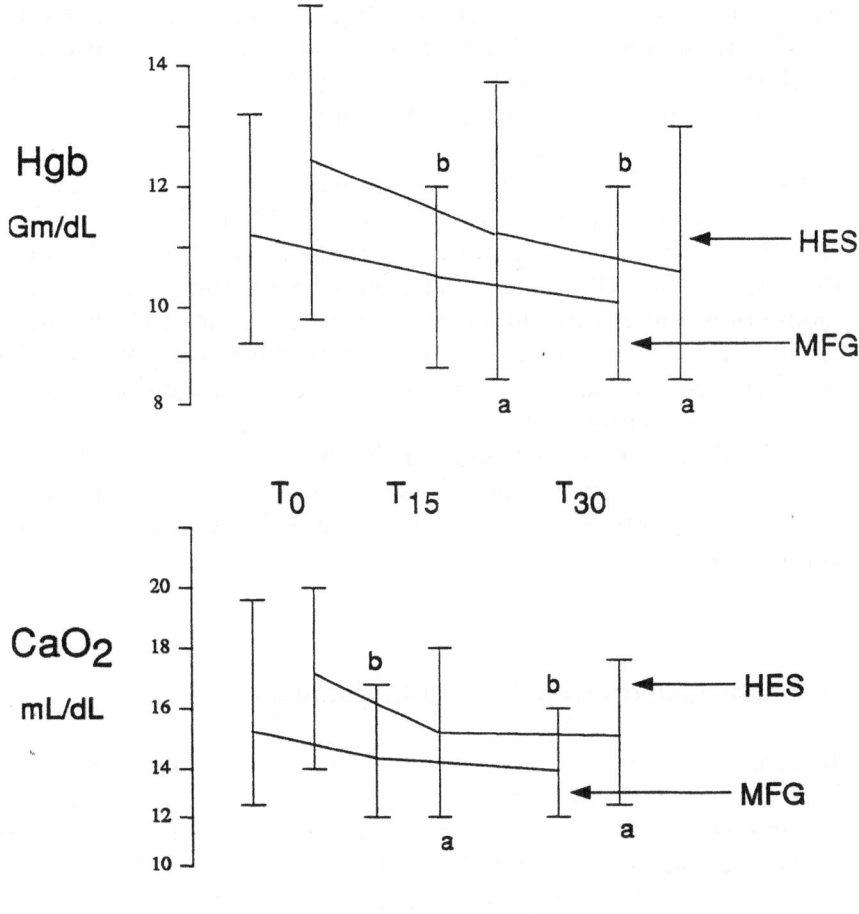

a = p <0.01, b = p <0.05 compared to T_0

Fig. 2.7

similar there was more significant haemodilution in the pentastarch group such that mean CaO_2 fell from 14.0 ml/dl to 10.9 ml/
dl and DO_2 from 364 to 336 ml/min/m^2 whereas the haemodiluting effect of albumin was much less so that mean DO_2 increased
from 401 to 457 ml/min/m^2 (these results calculated from the data
provided in the original report). Our group recently compared the
effects of MFG to those of high molecular weight HES in a randomised, non-crossover study in a group of patients with severe

ARDS most of whom were septic [35]. The cardiorespiratory effects of rapid infusion of 0.5 l of each solution were recorded at baseline (T0), 15 min (T15) and 30 min (T30). No other change in therapy was undertaken during this period. The results are summarised in Figs. 2.5–2.7.

The greater haemodiluting effect of HES was shown by decreases in CaO_2 from 17±3.2 ml/dl to 15±2.8 ml/dl compared to 15.3±2.6 ml/dl to 14.1±2.2 ml/dl in response to MFG. The poor CO response to HES meant that coupled with the degree of haemodilution there was no significant increase in DO_2 although PAOP and MAP all increased. Once again, there was poor correlation between CVP and PAOP at all recorded times and changes in CVP were not significant.

It should be noted that none of the studies cited above (or any others in the literature) have shown a worsening of the degree of pulmonary insufficiency in response to volume expansion with colloid solutions.

Traumatic Rhabdomyolysis – Crush Syndrome

In contradistinction to major trauma this is a situation which can be managed on clinical grounds in the vast majority of cases. It is an important syndrome because initial management based on an understanding of the pathophysiology can salvage a patient from a potentially lethal injury. It is generally accepted that the first formal description of this syndrome was by Bywaters [36], who described the sequence of events occurring in civilian victims of air raids in London during World War II. The classic course of events was rescue with injuries apparently confined to the lower limbs followed within hours by circulatory collapse, hyperkalaemia, uraemia, cardiac arrest and death. Bywaters also described prevention of this problem by adequate volume loading. In actual fact, in retrospect, some of the cases described by Cannon [7] were suffering from this syndrome and the method of experimental injury produced by Blalock [9] almost certainly mimicked this syndrome in the laboratory. The pathophysiology is related to an initial compression (crush) injury, which may of itself be unimpressive. This probably leads to breakdown of the sarcolemmal Na^+/K^+ pump and loss of efflux of Ca^{2+} from the cell leading to intracellular hypercalcaemia which further disrupts muscle fibres. The intramuscular pressure in trapped limbs may be greater than 200 mm Hg in less than 60 min and massive rhabdomyolysis can occur without classic signs of ischaemia. Ultimately intracompartmental pressure may exceed perfusion pressure and lead to further rhabdomyolysis. The release of intracellular muscle contents occurs after extrication of the victim. There is an immediate cascade of biochemical abnormalities (Table 2.7).

This coincides with sudden hypovolaemia related to release of the tourniquet effect of the entrapment pressure. Myoglobin is rapidly nephrotoxic by a complex series of mechanisms which are generally dependent on its precipitation in renal tubules [37]. This is exacerbated by the high urate load – so metabolic acidosis, hyperkalaemia, hypocalcaemia, anuria and hypovolaemia occur simultaneously with disastrous results [38].

Volume replacement should begin as soon as possible and preferably prior to extrication. A reasonable regime would be to give at least 1.5–2 l of an isotonic solution containing Na^+ (*not* normal saline, see below) or 1.0 l of MFG during the rescue – this for the trapped limb(s) alone, the presence of other injuries would obviously govern the need for additional fluids. After rescue volume requirements may be enormous (up to 12 l/day of crystalloid). An initial diuresis of 8 l/day has been advocated and should be maintained until myoglobinuria disappears [38]. In addition to mannitol to promote the diuresis, supplemental $NaHCO_3^-$ is usually re-

Table 2.7. Consequences of acute rhabidomyolysis

Hypovolemia
Metabolic acidosis
Hyperkalemia
Raised serum creatinine
Hyperuricemia
Hyperphosphatemia
Hypocalcemia
Myoglobinemia/uria
Raised creatinine phosphokinase

Table 2.8. Characteristics of six patients with traumatic rhabdomyolysis

Patient	Age	ISS	CPK^M	[K+]^i	Creatinine^M	pH	pH	S/N
1	17	24	65,000	5.8	480	7.25	5	S
2	26	16	136,000	5.2	620	7.30	5	S
3	42	32	200,000	7.2	360	7.12	5	S
4	22	28	86,000	6.5	840	7.05	5	S
5	56	38	180,000	4.9	520	7.32	5	NS
6	33	42	140,000	8.8	4.10	7.22	5	S

quired to maintain urine pH as near to neutral as possible to prevent precipitation of myoglobin and uric acid which are both highly insoluble in acidic tubular fluid [37]. The data for six patients arranged according to this regime are shown in Table 2.8.

Our own experience with earthquake victims in Armenia and Iran (unpublished data) suggests that this simple approach is under-utilised as it may be in western countries. Two patients in the above series have been transferred from other hospitals for dialysis which was not needed after initiation of the regime described above.

Post-operative Shock

Hypotension following emergency or elective surgery can be due to a variety of causes including sepsis, myocardial ischaemia or infarction, pulmonary embolism or adverse reaction to anaesthetic agents. However, hypovolaemia is common even after apparently uncomplicated and well controlled surgical procedures. In a clinical study Shires [39] demonstrated, using radio-isotope techniques, that, for instance, elective gastrectomy or cholecystectomy was associated with a 5–10 l deficit in extracellular fluid volume even when visible fluid and blood loss had been corrected. This occult loss he proposed was due to sequestration of fluid into bowel, peritoneum and the wound. He coined the term third space as a name for this hidden compartment and this term has gained universal acceptance.

We prospectively studied 50 patients who were transferred to the ICU after successful repair of a ruptured abdominal aortic aneurysm [40]. In contradistinction to the work by Bland and Shoemaker [41] we found that no O_2T variable was predictive of survival or non-survival. There were only three physiological differences between survivors and non-survivors – PAOP, arterial blood lactate, and core temperature.

Cardiogenic Shock

Even in the thrombolytic era the incidence of cardiogenic shock following acute myocardial infarction (AMI) remains 5%–10% of cases [42]. The O_2T patterns found in cardiogenic shock resemble those seen in resuscitated trauma with a critically low DO_2, S_VO_2 and very high OER [43] (Fig. 2.8).

A classic study by Forrester showed that at least 25% of cases of shock following AMI were associated with a low PAOP and that volume therapy might be appropriate in such cases – even when there was clinical evidence of pulmonary oedema [44] – a concept that many cardiologists find difficult to grasp.

A more recent study by our group [45] showed that the majority of cases of shock following AMI without true cardiogenic pulmonary oedema were associated with the surface ECG pattern of

OXYGEN TRANSPORT PATTERNS IN CARDIOGENIC SHOCK

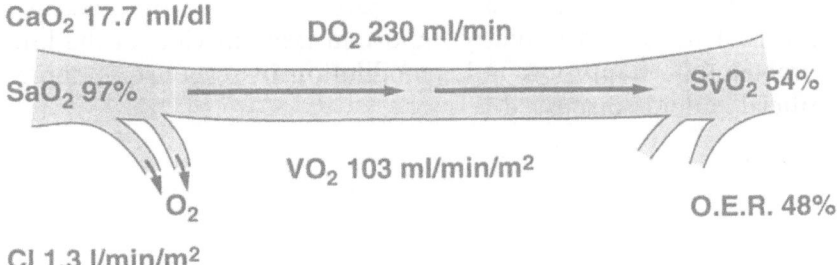

CaO$_2$ 17.7 ml/dl   DO$_2$ 230 ml/min

SaO$_2$ 97%   S$\bar{v}$O$_2$ 54%

VO$_2$ 103 ml/min/m^2

O$_2$ O.E.R. 48%

CI 1.3 l/min/m^2

Fig. 2.8

inferior myocardial infarction and clinical and haemodynamic evidence of right ventricular infarction. However, even in these cases, for a variety of reasons hypoxaemia is common and often unresponsive to increases in inspired O_2 concentration. It is important to realise that the most striking physical signs as far as the cardiologist may be concerned, elevated jugular venous pressure, right ventricular third heart sound, for instance, are not the cause unless diuretic or vasodilator therapy has been inappropriately used. The low CO seen in these cases is associated with reduced LVSWI, and if shock improves in response to therapy it is associated with significant increases in left ventricular not right ventricular function [46]. Most authorities now agree that shock following AMI must be addressed by some form of myocardial revascularisation – probably perivenous angioplasty or by-pass grafting.

Optimal Haematocrit

This is a controversial subject with experts holding widely differing opinions. Indeed, two reviews have recently been published with widely differing conclusions and recommendations. Van der Linden concluded that no firm conclusion on the actual level of Hb concentration or blood haematocrit could be made and each patient should be assessed individually especially with regard to the ability of CO to increase to compensate for reduced CaO_2. However, Spahn and Pasch took a differing standpoint but concentrated on studies of elective surgical patients. Sibbald has recently summarised powerful data to show that the Hb concentration should be maintained at a normal level in the presence of sepsis. This is a particularly important issue in view of the known problems of inappropriate haemodilution in response to some artificial colloids discussed.

Better Clinical Guidelines: The Shock Index?

As discussed previously repeated studies have shown a poor correlation between clinical assessment of adequacy of volume replacement and objective measurements of left ventricular pre-load or blood volume in patients who ultimately require ICU admission. Obviously not all such will require invasive monitoring and even in patients with the severest injuries or burns it is impractical as an immediate procedure in the emergency department. Is there any way in which the vital signs can be interpreted in a different manner so as to give the referring clinician an improved insight into the status of volume replacement in relation to adequacy of DO_2? A surprisingly simple and convenient calculation seems to have been overlooked, rather sadly it seems, because the original description was published in German. The shock index was originally described by Allgower and Buri in 1967 [46]. The shock index is the ratio of heart rate to systolic blood pressure:

Shock index=Heart rate/Systolic BP

The original authors observed a normal value of 0.5–0.7 which increased to a maximum of 2.5 during acute gastrointestinal haemorrhage. As described above individual values of heart rate and mean arterial blood pressure have been shown to be a poor indicator of volume status. We recently re-evaluated the shock index [47] in clinical septic shock and in experimental haemorrhagic shock in anaesthetised pigs as part of an ongoing study into the effects of nociceptive stimulation on the critical level of DO_2. In septic shock as expected there was no clear-cut relationship between DO_2, VO_2 and shock index but a good correlation (r=−0.68, Pearson correlation coefficient, p<0.01) with LVSWI. In experimental haemorrhagic shock there was an excellent correlation in individual animals between shock index and critical DO_2 – below which oxygen consumption (VO_2) fell as lactate levels rose (Fig. 2.8).

The correlation with SVI and DO_2 was significant at −0.82 and −0.62 respectively (p<0.01). We applied the shock index retrospectively to the data of Cournand, which represents one of the few, or possibly the only, study of haemodynamic and oxygen transport variables in untreated haemorrhagic and hypovolemic shock in humans. There was, once again, a close inverse correlation between shock index and VO_2 ($r=-0.76$, $p<0.01$). Further studies are in progress but the available data are very suggestive that use of the shock index may provide a better guide to management of hypovolaemic shock than individual consideration of heart rate and blood pressure or their trends.

Physicochemical Properties of Artificial Colloids

The physicochemical properties of individual artificial colloids have been grossly neglected by clinicians and the potential effects of these on resuscitation seem to have been completely ignored by manufacturers and investigators.

The clinical properties of relevance include the concentrations of monovalent ions (sodium, potassium, bicarbonate, and chloride), divalent ions (calcium, magnesium, sulphate) and trivalent ions (e.g. phosphate). Another important consideration is the pH of the solution. Physical properties of importance are the relative viscosity, gel point and colloid osmotic pressure. For instance two gelatin solutions are routinely used in Europe and clinicians tend to regard them as identical. However, a comparison of the properties of the two based on information supplied by the manufacturers reveals striking differences.

Another physical variable which is misunderstood and neglected by clinicians is the polydispersity ratio of these solutions. This is the ratio of weight average to number average of the estimated molecular weights of the solutions. For albumin, in which all molecules are of identical size, this ratio is 1. In the case of artificial colloids the most desirable ratio is that of dextran 40. However, the use of this is severely limited by its nephrotoxicity. Gelatins are for practical purposes the most desirable artificial colloid in this regard.

Summary and Conclusions

1. Artificial colloids should not be considered as interchangeable as they have differing physicochemical and physiological properties.
2. In all forms of shock there is a tendency for clinicians to under-estimate the volume deficit of their patients.
3. Monitoring of CVP is dangerous in critically ill patients and should be abandoned.

References

1. Edwards JD, Whittaker S, Prior A (1986) Cardiogenic shock without a critically elevated left ventricular end diastolic pressure: management and outcome in eighteen patients. Brit Heart J 55:549–553
2. Vincent J-L, Weil MH, Puri V, Carlson RW (1981) Circulatory shock associated with purulent peritonitis. Am J Surg 142:262–270
3. Rady MY, Edwards JD, Nightingale P (1992) Early cardiorespiratory findings after severe blunt thoracic trauma and their relation to outcome. Br J Surg 79:6568
4. Cournand A, Riley RL, Bradley SE et al. (1943) Studies of the circulation in clinical shock. Surgery 13:964–995
5. Haupt MT (1993) Therapy: Effects of Fluid Resuscitation In: Edwards JD, Shoemaker WC, Vincent J-L (eds) Oxygen transport principles and practice. Balli're Tindall, London. pp 175–192
6. Rady MY, Nightingale P, Little RA, Edwards JD (1992) Shock index: a re-evaluation in circulatory failure. Resuscitation 23:227–234
7. Cannon WB (1918) A consideration of the nature of wound shock. JAMA 70:611–617
8. Cannon WB, Fraser J, Cowell EM (1918) The preventive treatment of wound shock. JAMA 70:68–621
9. Blalock A.(1929) Experimental shock: The cause of the low blood pressure produced by muscle injury. Arch Surg 20:959–996
10. Edwards JD, Redmond AD, Nightingale P, Wilkins RG (1988) Oxygen consumption following trauma: a reappraisal in severely injured patients requiring mechanical ventilation. Br J Surg 75:690–692
11. Moore FA, Haenel JB, Moore E, Whitehill TA (1992) Commensurate oxygen consumption in response to maximal oxygen availability predicts post-injury multiple organ failure. J Trauma 33:58–67
12. Fleming A, Bishop M, Shoemaker WC, Appel P, Sufficool W, Kuvhenguwha A, Kennedy F, Chai-Jun Wo (1992) Prospective trial of supranormal

values as goals in resuscitation in severe trauma. Arch Surg 127:1175–1181

13. Advanced Trauma Life Support (1994) Comm Trauma, American College of Surgeons. E Erie St, Chicago

14. Simmons RS, Berdine GG, Seidenfield JJ, Prihoda TJ, Harris GD, Smith JD, Gilbert J, Mota E, Johanson Jr, WG (1987) Fluid balance and the adult respiratory distress syndrome. Am Rev Respir Dis 135:924–929

15. Schuller D, Mitchell JP, Calandrino, Schuster DP (1991) Fluid balance during pulmonary edema. Is fluid a marker or a cause of poor outcome? Chest 100:1068–1075

16. Snajder J, Wood D (1991) Beneficial effects of reducing pulmonary oedema in Patients with acute hypoxemic respiratory failure. Chest 100:890–891

17. Asbaugh DG, Bigelow DB, Petty TL, Levine BE (1967) Acute respiratory distress in adults. Lancet ii:319–323

18. Pepe PE, Potkin RT, Reus DH, Hudson LD, Carrico CJ (1982) Clinical predictors of the Adult Respiratory Distress Syndrome. Am J Surg 144:124–130

19. Shoemaker WC, Appel P, Czer LSC, Bland R, Schwartz S, Hopkins JA (1980) Pathogenesis of respiratory failure (ARDS) after haemorrhage and trauma. Crit Care Med 8:504–512

20. Montgomery AB, Stager MA, Carrico J, Hudson LD (1985) Causes of mortality in patients with the adult respiratory distress syndrome. Am Rev Respir Dis 132:485–489

21. Villar J, Manzaur J, Blazquez M, Quintana J, Lubillo S (1991) Multiple system organ failure in acute respiratory failure. J Crit Care 2:75–80

22. Russel J, Ronco J, Lockhat D, Belzberg A, Kiess M, Dodek P (1990) Oxygen delivery and consumption and ventricular preload are greater in survivors than in non survivors of the Adult Respiratory Distress Syndrome. Am Rev Respir Dis 141:659–665

23. O'Keefe N, Clarke C, Edwards JD (1993) Cardiorespiratory variables in severe ARDS in relation to outcome. Crit Care Med 21:S209(A)

24. Chadwick S, Edwards JD, Nightingale P(1993) The adequacy of volume replacement in trauma victims prior to admission to Intensive Care. Crit Care Med 21:S246

25. Dries DJ, Waxman K (1991) Adequate resuscitation of burns may not be measured by urine output and vital signs. Crit Care Med 327–329

26. Millar JG, Bunting P, Burd DAR, Edwards JD (1994) Early cardiorespiratory patterns in patients with major burns and pulmonary insufficiency. Burns 20:542–546

27. Shoemaker WC (1976) Comparison of the relative effectiveness of whole blood transfusions and various types of fluid therapy in resuscitation. Crit Care Med 4:71–78

28. Shippy CR, Appel PL, Shoemaker WC (1984) Reliability of clinical monitoring to assess blood volume in critically ill patients. Crit Care Med 12:107–112

29. Haupt MT, Gilbert EM, Carlson RW (1985) Fluid loading increases oxygen consumption in septic patients with lactic acidosis. Am Rev Respir Dis 131:912–916

30. Gilbert EM, Haupt MT, Manadanas RY, Hauringa AJ, Carlson RW (1986) The effect of fluid loading, blood transfusion and catecholamine infusion on oxygen delivery and consumption in patients with sepsis. Am Rev Respir Dis 134:873–878

31. Manny J, Grindlinger GA, Dennis RC, et al. (1979) Myocardial performance curves as a guide to volume therapy. Surg Gynecol Obstet 149:863–873

32. Calvin JE, Dreiger AA, Sibbald WJ (1981) The haemodynamic effect of rapid fluid infusion in critically ill patients. Surgery 90:61–76

33. Edwards JD, Nightingale P, Wilkins RG, Faragher EB (1989) Haemodynamic and oxygen transport response to modified fluid gelatin in critically ill patients. Crit Care Med 17:996–998

34. Rackow EC, Falk JL, Fein A, et al. (1983) Fluid resuscitation in circulatory shock: a comparison of the cardiorespiratory effects of albumin, hetastarch, and slaine solutions in patients with hypovolemic and septic shock. Crit Care Med 11:839–850

35. Beards SC, Watts T, Edwards JD, Nightingale P, Faragher EB (1994) Comparison of the haemodynamic and oxygen transport responses to modified fluid gelatin and hetastarch in critically ill patients: A randomized trial. Crit Care Med 22:600–605

36. Bywaters EGL, Beall D (1941) Crush injuries with impairment of renal function. Br Med J 1:427–432

37. Zager RA (1989) Studies of mechanisms and protective maneuvers in myoglobinuric acute renal injury. Lab Invest 60:619–629

38. Better S, Stein JH (1990) Early management of shock and prophylaxis of acute renal failure in traumatic rhabdomylosis. N Engl J Med 332:825–829

39. Shires PT, Williams J, Brown F (1961) Acute changes in extracellular fluids associated with major surgical procedures. 154:803–810

40. Parry A, Edwards JD (1995) Cardiorespiratory variables after repair of rupture abdominal aortic aneursym. Crit Care Med S3

41. Bland RD, Shoemaker WC, Abraham E, Cobo JC (1985) Hemodynamic and oxygen transport patterns in surviving and non surviving postoperative patients. Crit Care Med 13:85–90

42. Gheorghiade M, Ruzumna P, Borzak S, Havstad S, Ali A, Goldstein S (1996) Decline in the rate of hospital mortality from acute myocardial infarction: impact of changing management strategies. Am Heart J 131:250–256

43. Creamer JE, Edwards JD, Nightingale P (1990) Hemodynamic and oxygen transport variables in cardiogenic shock secondary to acute myocardial infarction, and response to treatment. Am J Cardiol 65:1297–1300

44. Forrester JS, Diamond GA, Swan HJC (1977) Correlative classification of clinical and hemodynamic function after acute myocardial infarction. Am J Cardiol 39:137
45. Edwards JD, Whittaker S, Prior A (1986) Cardiogenic shock without a critically elevated left ventricular end diastolic pressure: management and outcome in eighteen patients. Brit Heart J 55:549–553
46. Creamer JE, Edwards JD, Nightingale P (1991) Mechanism of shock associated with right ventricular infarction. Br Heart J 65:63–67

CHAPTER 3

Which Hydroxyethyl Starch for Which Indication?

3

G. AUDIBERT, M.C. LAXENAIRE

Plasma substitutes are widely used to maintain circulatory dynamics during various types of shock. Plasma volume can be expanded with several types of colloids, belonging to four pharmacological families: gelatins, dextrans, starches, and albumin. Rather than attempting to determine which type of solution is superior to others, we consider it appropriate to outline the proper role of each in the context of its specific indications and characteristics. This chapter defines advantages and side effects of the use of starches in treating hypovolemia. Factors that are discussed include blood volume expanding efficiency, hemostasis impairment, allergic reactions, and the effect on microcirculation. Finally, indications are suggested for various clinical situations.

Starch Characteristics

Hemodynamic Effects of HES

Starches are chemically modified polymers composed of polysaccharide molecules, derivatives of amylopectine, i.e., they are of vegetal origin. This is in contrast to gelatins, which are composed of polypeptide molecules obtained after bovine collagen hydrolysis, i.e., they are of animal origin. However, in 1996 the European Medicine Evaluation Agency published its view that medical products containing gelatin are safe regarding the transmission of bovine spongiform encephalopathy.

The major characteristics of several plasma volume expanders are summarized in Table 3.1. Hydroxyethyl starches (HES) are

Table 3.1. Plasma volume expanders characteristics

	Initial plasma volume expansion (%)	Duration of efficacy (h)	Hemostatic competence	Colloid osmotic pressure (mmHg)
HES 6%/200/0.6	100–140	12–18	↓	32
HES 6%/200/0.5	100–140	4–8	↓	32
Pentastarch 10%/200	140–170	6–8	↓	55
Hetastarch 6%/400	80–100	12–24	↓↓	28
Gelatin 3%	60–80	3–5	→	–
Dextran 10%/40	170–180	4–6	↓↓	–
Dextran 6%/60	100	6–8	↓↓	58
Albumin 4%	70–80	6–8	→	22

polymers containing mixtures of differently sized molecules, ranging from small molecules which may leak from the intravascular space to large molecules that may impair blood coagulation [1]. An HES with a mean molecular weight (MW) of 450 kDa is classified as high-MW whereas an HES with mean MW of 200 kDa is classified as a medium-MW HES. The higher the MW, the greater is the plasma volume expansion. Under normal capillary permeability conditions larger molecules (more than 65 kDa) are retained in the intravascular space where they generate colloid osmotic pressure. The colloid osmotic pressure of a plasma expander is of great importance for its initial plasma volume expanding capacity. This explains why medium-MW HES has an initial plasma volume expanding capacity in excess of the infused volume (Table 3.1) [2].

However, among the medium-MW HES a higher substitution value (0.6) is responsible for a prolonged volume-supporting capacity. This long-lasting effect may be considered as an advantage, but high substitution may also have important drawbacks. In vivo, HES molecules are cleaved by serum amylase to residues that are eventually eliminated by the kidney. However, the HES solution, especially if initial substitution is high, contains some molecules with very a high substitution value (>0.7), which prevents amylase cleavage and therefore renal excretion. The breakdown rate may also be influenced by the C2/C6 hydroxyethylation ratio [3]. All this may lead to long intravascular persistence. HES plasma levels have been shown to remain still detectable 35 days after infusion of 500 ml 10% HES 200/0.5 [4]. HES 200/0.5 has been found to persist in lymph nodes and muscle biopsies for as long as 10 months after a dose of 1 g/kg body weight [5]. This phenomenon may account for the intense itching reported by patients receiving HES infusion [6]. In contrast, dextrans and gelatins are fully metabolized to carbon dioxide and water.

HES and Hemostasis

It is generally thought that HES solutions interfere with normal hemostasis. The risk is particularly high with high-MW HES. Principally the primary hemostasis is affected, leading to von Willebrand-like syndrome and impairment of platelet functions. In patients undergoing coronary surgery a mean volume of 840 ml HES 450 has been found responsible for a decrease in platelet aggregation, leading to an increase in post-bypass blood loss (890 ml vs. 660 ml in patients receiving HES/200/0.5) [7]. The infusion of medium-MW HES did not affect coagulation parameters.

Nevertheless recent data indicate that even medium-MW HES may impair hemostasis. In patients receiving a daily infusion of 500 ml HES 200/0.6 for 10 days, a sharp decrease was found in von Willebrand antigen at the end of the treatment [8]. This was related to an increase in HES serum concentration after 10 days – with HES 200/0.6 but not with HES 200/0.5. There was no instance of bleeding complication in this study. However, in a study including 42 patients scheduled for total hip replacement and randomized to receive infusion of either HES 200/0 or gelatin, a volume of 28 ml/kg HES 200/0.5 was found to be associated with significant increased blood loss [9]; however, the volume of packed red cell transfusions was slightly greater in the gelatin group. After HES four patients were found to have an abnormal bleeding time. Therefore the debate on the clinical relevance of HES-induced hemostasis impairment is still open.

HES and Allergic Reactions

All colloids used for plasma volume support may induce anaphylactoid reactions. Data from large prospective studies suggest that the risk associated with HES is low (Table 3.2). A multicenter French survey of more than 15,000 patients reported the risk associated with HES to be 0.058% (per patient) [10]. HES was found to be the safest plasma expander regarding anaphylactoid reaction risk. The allergic reaction rate was a slightly higher than in the classical Ring and Messmer study [11], but it must be pointed out that the reactions rate was reported by patients in the French study and by units in the German study.

HES and Microcirculation

Plasma substitutes may be used to improve blood rheology. In animals dextran 40 and HES have been shown to induce the most beneficial rheological effects [12]. In humans there have been only few comparative studies. One of these included 50 patients undergoing preoperative hemodilution [13], randomized to receive either 4% albumin, 3.5% dextran 40, gelatin, or HES 200/0.62. Ten patients without hemodilution were chosen as controls. HES did not alter blood viscosity, but this was decreased after albumin and dextran. Erythrocyte aggregation was markedly decreased after al-

Table 3.2. Incidence of anaphylactoid reactions with plasma expanders

	% units [11]	% patients [10]
HES	0.085	0.058
Gelatin		
Urea linked	0.146	0.852
Modified fluid	0.066	0.325
Dextran		
40	0.007	0.269
60/75	0.069	0.286
Albumin	0.011	0.099

bumin and dextran but was unchanged after HES. These findings suggest that if albumin and dextran are considered as the substitutes of choice for improving rheological conditions, HES can be regarded as relatively neutral for rheological effects.

Clinical Indications of HES

Preoperative Hemodilution

Preoperative hemodilution has become widely used to avoid transfusion-transmitted diseases. To replace the withdrawn blood volume the plasma volume expanding capacity of the colloid must be long enough to prevent a rebound of hypovolemia in the postoperative period. HES has been shown to achieve this goal. In a study including 18 patients scheduled for abdominal aortic surgery HES 200/0.6 maintained mean arterial pressure, cardiac index, and blood volume during the first postoperative 24 h [14]. In orthopedic surgery 7 h after the hemodilution 76% of the infused HES volume was still intravascular, as compared with 56% of an infused gelatin volume [9]. These results confirm that HES is suitable for preoperative hemodilution.

Perioperative Blood Loss Replacement

Maintaining peri- and postoperative normovolemia is of utmost importance for limiting morbidity and mortality after surgery. HES may be used until a trigger hemoglobin value is reached for homologous transfusion, determined specifically for each patient. In 40 patients undergoing elective abdominal aortic surgery 5% HES 450 was found as effective as 5% albumin for maintaining hemodynamics [15]. Blood transfusions were identical in both groups, as well as hemostasis parameters. Nevertheless, since large volumes of HES may impair hemostatic function and therefore increase the risk of bleeding, the maximal recommended amount of infused HES is 33 ml/kg per 24 h.

HES and Pregnancy

In France artificial colloids cannot be used during pregnancy. Both dextrans and gelatins have been involved in severe allergic reactions of the fetus or of the mother. When HES was released onto the French market, the above contraindication was extended to HES although no severe allergic reactions were reported in pregnant women. However, in other European countries, HES are allowed during pregnancy. Cristalloids can be used for blood loss less than 1000 ml [16]; colloids must be infused above this threshold.

HES in Shock States

Experimental studies have shown potential beneficial effects of HES in shock states. In a model of rat limb ischemia-reperfusion injury medium-MW HES was found to decrease water content more than dextran or low-MW HES [17]. These results suggest that medium-MW HES is able to reduce abnormal microvascular permeability. In vitro, HES 450 but not albumin has been shown to inhibit endothelial activation, which can prevent neutrophil adherence during sepsis syndrome [18]. In a mouse model of hemorrhage HES 450 restored macrophage activation integrity and prevented increase in circulating interleukin 6 level [19].

Clinical studies have confirmed the hemodynamic efficacy of HES in patients suffering from shock. HES 450 was compared with gelatin in 28 patients with hypovolemia, ventilated for acute respiratory failure [20]; in both groups mean arterial pressure, cardiac index, stroke volume increased. However, the results of this study were reported only for the first 30 min. In 30 trauma patients and 30 septic patients 10% HES 200 was compared with 20% albumin and cardiorespiratory variables for 5 days [21]. Cardiac index increased only in the HES group (both in trauma and septic patients). Right ventricular ejection fraction increased in the HES group. Gastric mucosal pH remained normal in the HES group and decreased in septic patients receiving albumin. The same investigators have shown that in septic patients treatment with HES limits the increase in adhesion molecules whereas with albumin the plasma concentration of these molecules increases [22].

HES and Head Trauma

In patients with head trauma plasma volume expansion may increase cerebral edema, with a simultaneous increase in intracranial pressure. In this situation HES may seem a good choice because of its high osmolarity and colloid osmotic pressure. When compared with normal or hypertonic saline, HES has been found safe and not to increase intracranial pressure in animals receiving a volume of 20 ml/kg [23].

HES in Brain-Dead Donors

After brain death hypovolemia is a common finding because of diabetes insipidus and loss of sympathetic tone. Hemodynamic maintenance is a key point for organ preservation. HES administered in this situation has been suggested to be responsible for renal function impairment. A prospective randomized study of 27 brain dead donors found plasma volume expansion with HES 200/ 0.6 and with gelatin. Kidney recipients were followed for 6 weeks. In the HES group more patients required initial extrarenal hemodialysis or hemofiltration [24]. During the first 10 days serum creatinine concentration was significantly lower in the gelatin group. Interestingly, renal biopsies were obtained in several patients in the HES group, showing osmotic nephrosis-like lesions in the tubules. However, no information was given regarding the delayed graft function and graft survival.

References

1. Arfors KE, Buckley PB (1997) Pharmacological characteristics of artificial colloids. Clin Anaesthesiol 11 (1):15–47

2. Haljamae H, Dahlquist M, Walentin F (1997) Artificial colloids in clinical practice: pros and cons. Clin Anaesthesiol 11 (1):49–79
3. Treib J, Haass A, Pindur G, Seyfert UT, Treib W, Grauer MT, Jung F, Wenzel E, Schimrigk K (1995) HES 200/0.5 is not HES 200/0.5. Influence of the C2/C6 hydroxyethylation ratio of hydroxyethylstarch (HES) on hemorheology coagulation and elimination kinetics. Thromb Haemost 74:1452–1456
4. Kohler H, Zschiedrich H, Linfante A (1982) The elimination of HES 200/0.5, dextran 40 and oxypolygelatine. Klin Wochenschr 60:293–301
5. Sirtl C, Hubner G, Jesch F (1988) Zur Speicherung von hoch und mittel-molekularer Hydroxyäthylstärke (HÄS) in meuschlichen Gewebe. Beitr Anaesthesiol Intens Med 26:74–97
6. Spittal MJ, Findlay GP (1995) The seven year itch. Anaesthesia 50:913–914
7. Boldt J, Knothe C, Zickmann B, Andres P, Dopper F, Hempelmann G (1993) Influence of different intravascular volume therapies on platelet function in patients undergoing cardiopulmonary bypass. Anesth Analg 76:1185–1190
8. Treib J, Haass A, Pindur G, Grauer MT, Wenzel E, Schimrigk K (1996) All medium starches are not the same: influence of the degree of hydroxyethyl substitution of hydroxyethyl starch on plasma volume, hemorrheologic conditions and coagulation. Transfusion 36:450–455
9. Mortelmans YJ, Kermant G, Verbruggen AM, Arnout JM, Vermylen J, van Aken H, Mortelmans LA (1995) Effects of 6% hydroxyethylstarch and 3% modified fluid gelatin on intravascular volume and coagulation during intraoperative hemodilution. Anesth Analg 81:1235–1242
10. Laxenaire MC, Charpentier C, Feldman L (1994) Anaphylactoid reactions to colloid plasma substitutes: frequency, risk factors, mechanisms. A French prospective multicentre inquiry. Ann Fr Anesth Reanim 13:301–310
11. Ring J, Messmer K (1977) Incidence and severity of anaphylactoid reactions to colloid volume substituts. Lancet I:466–469
12. Goto Y, Sakakura S, Hatta M (1985) Hemorheological effects of colloid plasma substitutes infusion. A comparative study. Acta Anaesthesiol Scand 29:217–223
13. Audibert G, Donner M, Lefevre JC, Stoltz JF, Laxenaire MC (1994) Rheologic effects of plasma substitutes used for preoperative hemodilution. Anesth Analg 78:740–745
14. Baron JF, de Kegel D, Prost AC, Mundler PO, Arthaud M, Basset G (1991) Low molecular weight hydroethylstarch 6% compared to albumin 4% during intentional hemodilution. Intensive Care Med 17:141–148
15. Gold MS, Russo J, Tissot M, Weinhouse G, Riles T (1990) Comparison of hetastarch to albumin for perioperative bleeding in patients undergoing abdominal aortic aneurysm surgery. A prospective, randomized study. Ann Surg 211:482–485
16. Knippel RA, Hatangadi SB (1995) Acute hypotension related to hemorrhage in the obstetric patient. Obstet Gynecol Clin North Am 22:111–129

17. Zikria BA, Subbarto C, Oz MC, Shih ST, MacLeod PF, Sachdev R, Freeman HP, Hardy MA (1989) Macromolecules reduce abnormal microvascular permeability in rat limb ischemia-reperfusion injury. Crit Care Med 17:1306–1309
18. Collis RE, Collins PW, Gutteridge CN, Kaul A, Newland AC, Williams DM, Webb AR (1994) The effect of hydroxyethylstarch and other plasma substitutes on endothelial cell activation; an in vitro study. Intensive Care Med 20:37–41
19. Schmand JF, Ayala A, Morrison MH, Chaudry IH (1995) Effects of hydroxyethylstarch after trauma-hemorrhagic shock: restoration of macrophage integrity and prevention of increased circulating interleukin 6 levels. Crit Care Med 23:806–814
20. Beards SC, Watt T, Edwards JD, Nightingale P, Farragher EB (1994) Comparison of the hemodynamic and oxygen transport responses to modified fluid gelatin and hetastarch in critically ill patients: a prospective, randomized trial. Crit Care Med 22:600–605
21. Boldt J, Heesen M, Müller M, Pabsdorf M, Hempelmann G (1996) The effects of albumin versus hydroxyethyl starch solution on cardiorespiratory variables in critically ill patients. Anesth Analg 83:254–261
22. Boldt J, Müller M, Heesen M, Neumann K, Hempelmann G (1996) Influence of different volume therapies and pentoxifylline infusion on circulating soluble adhesion molecules variables in critically ill patients. Crit Care Med 24:385–391
23. Ducey JP, Mozingo DW, Lamiell JM, Okerburg C, Gueller GE (1989) A comparison of the cerebral and cardiovascular resuscitation with isotonic and hypertonic saline, hetastarch and whole blood following hemorrhage. J Trauma 29:1510–1518
24. Cittanova ML, Leblanc I, Legendre CH, Mouquet C, Riou B, Coriat P (1996) Effect of hydroxyethylstarch in brain dead kidney donors on renal function in kidney transplant recipients. Lancet 348:1620–162

Volume Replacement Therapy with Dextrans: Are Dextrans Still Useful in Volume Replacement?

4

H. Litvan, J. I. Casas, J. M. Villar-Landeira

Dextrans in Volume Replacement Therapy

Dextran is a plasma volume expander introduced almost 50 years ago. It is a polysaccharide with a low degree of branching, produced by the fermentation of sucrose by the action of a bacteria, *Leuconostoc mesenteroides streptococus*, strain B512. By partial acid hydrolysis, most of the clinical dextrans are made with mean molecular weights (Mws) of 40,000 (dextran 40) or 70,000 daltons (dextran 70). In Table 4.1 some chemical characteristics of both clinical dextrans are compared to those of human albumin.

Dextran 40

Dextran 40, made up of particles having different molecular weights, has an average Mw of about 40,000 daltons, a molecular number (Mn) of 25,000 and a Mw/Mn ratio of 1.6 (compared with that of albumin, Mw/Mn = 1), monodisperse with all the particles with the same Mw: 69,000 daltons [1].

The 10% solution exerts a higher colloidal osmotic pressure than plasma proteins. With an oncotic capacity of 29–37 ml water/g dextran, it has a high water filtration capacity at the capillary bed. As the intravascular volume expands to a larger degree than the volume infused, the use of dextran requires the presence of mobile body water, or the intracellular compartment could become dehydrated. The volume expansion has a short effect (3–4 h) because of rapid renal excretion of the lower molecular weight dextran molecules. After intravenous infusion, about 60%–70% of

Table 4.1. Some chemical properties of clinical dextrans compared to human albumin [1, 2]

	Dextran 70 6%	Dextran 40 10%	Albumin 5%
Mw	70,000	40,000	69,000
Mn	35,000	25,000	69,000
Mw/Mn	2.0	1.6	1
Oncotic capacity (ml/g)	25–29	29–37	18–20

Mw, molecular weight (weight average) daltons; Mn, molecular weight (number average).

the product is excreted in the urine in the first 12 h [2]. As noted above, dextran 40 should not be used in dehydrated patients, and it no longer plays a role as a plasma volume expander.

Dextran 70

Dextran 70 has an average Mw of 70,000 daltons, a Mn of 35,000 and a Mw/Mn ratio of 2. As the oncotic capacity is Mw dependent, dextran 70 in a 6% solution exerts a colloidal osmotic pressure similar to that of plasma proteins, with an oncotic capacity of 23–29 ml water/g dextran [1].

After intravenous infusion, the volumetric effect persist about 6–8 h, the duration also being determined by the rate of renal excretion. Particles with Mws <50,000 daltons are excreted by the kidney, while particles with Mws >50,000 daltons are retained in the circulation and eliminated by biodegradation to glucose in the liver and other parenchymal cells. Some 12 h after the infusion only 30%–40% of the dextran is excreted in the urine [2].

Dextran 70 is an efficient plasma expander, providing an immediate and sustained volume support. Plasmatic volume expansion obtained with dextran 70 is greater than that obtained with equal volumes of isotonic albumin or gelatins and similar to that obtained with hydroxyethyl starch 200, 0.5 [3–6]. Also, the effect is as sustained as observed with albumin or hydroxyethyl starch (Table 4.2).

Table 4.2. Compared efficacy of standard colloids as plasma volume expanders [3–6]

	Volume expansion (%)	Volume effect (h)
Albumin 5%	100	6–8
Dextran 70 6%	100–150	6–8
HES* 200, 0.5 6%	100–140	6–8
Gelatins 3.5%	80–90	2–3

* HES, hydroxyethyl starch.

Other Indications

Other clinical indications for use of dextrans are: prolongation of the effects of hypertonic solutions, improvement of peripheral flow and as antithrombotic agents.

Prolongation of the Effects of Hypertonic Solutions

Hypertonic crystalloid solutions have been shown to be superior to normotonic solutions in terms of restoration of haemodynamic state, improving tissue perfusion and increasing survival of patients with traumatic shock. Small volumes of hypertonic solutions, up to 4 ml/kg body weight, were more efficient than four to ten times more isotonic crystalloids. As the effect of hypertonic solutions is very short, combined hypertonic hyperoncotic solutions have been used to obtain a more sustained effect [7].

A solution of 7.5% saline-dextran 70 6% has been shown to be highly effective in normalizing cardiovascular function in patients with haemorrhagic shock, due to rapid mobilization of fluid from the extravascular compartment [8]. This solution might also have other beneficial local factors, such as reversal of organ oedema, improvement of coronary blood supply, and a scavenging effect on toxic oxygen metabolites [9–11]. However, hypertonic dextran solutions can produce hyperosmolarity, hypernatremia, hypokalaemia and fluid overload.

This new clinical use of dextran is still being investigated as a form of therapy.

Improve Peripheral Flow

Both dextran 40 and dextran 70 could be used in conditions in which improved circulatory flow is required. While dextrans act principally by plasma volume expansion, they also produce a decrease in blood viscosity, which promotes a subsequent improvement in flow, and have a specific desegregating activity [2, 12]. For example, dextran 40 inhibits red blood cell aggregation and can be used to reduce blood viscosity in trauma patients, in whom microcirculatory blood flow deteriorates.

Funk and Baldinger [13] compared isovolemic exchange of blood (hematocrit 30%) with dextran or Ringer's solution and concluded that dextrans yielded hemodynamic stability and adequate tissue oxygen supply, whereas crystalloids alone jeopardized tissue perfusion and oxygenation.

Dextran has also been shown to form a very thick layer on the luminal surface of capillary endothelium, reducing the electrostatic charges. It may be that plasma flow could be facilitated by a reduced interaction of endothelial receptors with specific plasma proteins [14].

Antithrombotic Effect

Dextran can be used in the prophylaxis of postoperative thromboembolic disorders. An infusion of dextran on the third day after major trauma resulted in a decrease in fibrinolysis inhibitory activity to pretraumatic levels. Gruber et al. [15] compared dextran 70 and low-dose heparin in the prophylaxis of fatal postoperative pulmonary embolism. They found no statistically significant differences in the incidence of fatal pulmonary embolism. Moreover, fewer bleeding episodes but more allergic reactions were seen in the dextran group.

Dextran Side Effects

Renal failure, haemostatic disorders and allergic reactions have been described as dextran side effects. A relationship exists between the molecular weights of dextrans and their biological action as well as their side effects, both increasing with increasing molecular weight [2]. Dextrans with Mws > 200,000 daltons can interfere with blood coagulation, induce formation of circulating antibodies and result in more allergic reactions. To diminish these effects of clinical dextrans manufacturers have been careful not to permit the amount of particles with Mws > 115,000 daltons to exceed more than 10% [16]; however, molecules with Mw >250,000 daltons have been reported [17].

Renal Failure

An increase in renal plasma flow can be seen in normal volunteers after dextran infusion. However, the rapid renal excretion of dextran 40 in dehydrated patients with reduced urine flow can result in high urinary concentration which increases urinary viscosity and may cause oliguria and renal failure. Dextran low molecular weight particles are rapidly eliminated by the kidneys and their high oncotic efficiency can dehydrate the cells of the distal and proximal tubules. Dextran 40 is contraindicated in renal disease with oliguria. As stated by Twigley and Hillman [18] "...the damage is more likely to occur in just the condition where it would be used as a plasma volume expander, namely when renal perfusion is reduced."

Dextran 40 should not be used for volume replacement, but could be used for peripheral flow promotion, hypercoagulable states or ischaemic states [12]. By contrast, dextran 70 is not as rapidly excreted and does not cause renal effects.

Haemostatic Disorders

Dextran diminishes levels of factor VIII, platelet adhesiveness and increases thrombolysis.

Factor VIII reduction reaches its maximum effect 3–5 h after the infusion of dextran and can be reversed by the administration of factor VIII concentrate.

Table 4.3. Surgical bleeding patients (n = 27,346) at the Santa Creu i Sant Pau Hospital: 1994–1995

Blood loss (ml)	Surgical patients	(%)
<500	8219	77
500–1000	1814	17
1000–1000	427	4
>2000	214	2

Dextran also diminishes platelet adhesiveness. The thrombi formed in blood from dextran treated patients are significantly more lysable than thrombi from untreated patients [19]. Ljungström [20] has converted this negative effect of dextran into a positive one, using this activity as a prophylaxis against pulmonary embolism.

Bergqvist [21, 22] stated that dextran does not cause clinically relevant bleeding in doses less than 1–1.5 g/kg body weight. So, the suggested maximum dose as a plasma volume expander is 1.5 g/kg body weight by day. In order to increase the volume infused without reaching the maximum dose, dextran 60 3% has been introduced into the clinical setting [23].

Twigley and Hillman [18] have commented "We should measure the usefulness of a solution which is limited by an absolute and relatively small total dose in a clinical situation where an unpredictable intravascular volume has to be replaced." However, in a general hospital, the number of patients with non-controllable bleeding is small. Table 4.3 shows the number of surgical patients who had bleeding while at the Hospital Santa Creu i Sant Pau, a teaching general hospital in Barcelona, Spain. Some 39% of 27,346 surgical patients from 1994 to 1995 bled either during the operation or in post-operative intensive care; 11% were transfused, with fresh frozen plasma/red blood cells (ratio 0.08), that means very few units of plasma. Most of the patients bled less than 1000 ml. As only 2% of the patients bled more than 2000 ml, we could say that in our hospital dextran would be useful in at least 95% of surgical patients.

Dextran 70 is contraindicated in von Willebrand's disease and in patients with diminished platelet count.

Allergic Reactions

Many people have natural dextran-reactive antibodies, which may be induced by dextran itself or by cross-reactive microbial polysaccharides. Dextran is ingested as a regular contaminant of sucrose and is also produced by microorganisms of the gastrointestinal tract.

IgG class (mostly IgG2)-mediated anaphylaxis has been documented [24]. The incidence of severe allergic reactions during the 1970s was 0.022%, with 0.003% fatal reactions for dextran 40 and 0.004% for dextran 70 [25]. Fatal reactions occurred even after infusion of only 0.5–1 ml of dextran. For this reason the use of a 1 ml test-dose was strongly advised against. In 1982, by initial injection of hapten dextran (mean Mw 1000 daltons; dextran 1) considerable advances were made in the prevention of allergic reactions caused by dextran infusions [26]. Dextran 1 occupies the binding sites of dextran-reactive antibodies and prevents formation of large immune complexes with higher molecular weight dextrans, which may activate the complement system. Dextran 1 prevents severe anaphylactic reactions in a dose-dependent way. The recommended dose is 20 ml of a 15% solution by intravenous injection 1–2 min before infusion of the higher molecular weight dextran. The interval should not exceed 15 min and should be repeated if further infusions of dextran are required more than 48 h after the initial dose [26]. Dextran 1 does not reduce the incidence of mild reactions, which are not generally mediated by antibodies.

Comparing reports of severe anaphylactic reactions to dextran infusion during the period 1983–1992 (with prophylaxis with dextran 1) with reactions reported during the period 1975–1979 (without prophylaxis), Ljungström [27] found that the use of dextran 1 was associated with a 35-fold reduction in severe anaphylactic reactions to dextran infusion. The incidence fell from one severe reaction per 2000 patients to one per 70,000 patients. There were few adverse reactions to dextran 1, approximately one case per 100,000 doses; these were almost all mild, with minor clinical importance. The author also concluded that the introduction of hapten inhibition with dextran 1 dramatically reduces the risk of serious side effects caused by dextran, and suggested that dextran

Table 4.4. Evolution of dextran and other colloids used at the Santa Creu i Sant Pau Hospital: 1989 — 1996

Colloids[a]	1989 (%)	1996 (%)
Albumin 5%	2447 (23.3)	3221 (18.2)
Synthetic colloids	8055 (76.7)	14419 (81.7)
Dextran 70	1013 (9.6)	282 (1.6)
Dextran 40	256 (2)	69 (0.39)
Gelatins	6786 (64.6)	14068 (79.7)

[a] 500 ml bottles.

with hapten inhibition has possibly become the safest plasma substitute in current clinical use.

Evolution of the Use of Dextrans

In our hospital, as in the rest of Spain, dextran 1 is not available; thus there is diminished use of dextran. The evolution of dextran used at the Santa Creu i Sant Pau Hospital during 1989–1996 can be seen in Table 4.4. Dextran use fell from 12% of the colloids in 1989 to less than 2% in 1996, although during that period the use of colloids almost doubled. The largest increase was in the use of gelatins (from 65% to 80% of the total colloids used), while use of albumin fell from 23% to 18%. Hydroxyethyl starch 200, 0.5 was not introduced in Spain until 1997. Other countries, including England [17] and France [28], have also diminished the use of dextrans as plasma volume expander.

Conclusions

Dextran 70 has long been used as an efficient plasma volume expander. The incidence of side effects is low, principally involving allergic reactions, which are well known. While treatment with dextran 1 has considerably diminished the number of allergic reactions, it is not available in Spain; thus dextran 70 is not used as frequently as in the past.

References

1. Lutz H, Georgieff M (1986) Effects and side effects of colloid plasma substitutes as compared to albumin. Curr Stud Hematol Blood Transf 53:145–154
2. Lars Thorén (1981) The dextrans. Clinical data. In: Hennessen W (ed) Developments in biological standardization. Standardization of albumin, plasma substitutes and plasmapheresis. S. Karger, Basel, pp 157–167
3. Linko K, Mäkeläinen A (1988) Hydroxyethyl starch 120, dextran 70 and acetated Ringer's solution: hemodilution, albumin, colloid osmotic pressure and fluid balance following replacement of blood in pigs. Acta Anaesthesiol Scand 32:228–233
4. Lamke LO, Liljedahl SO (1976) Plasma volume changes after infusion of various plasma expanders. Resuscitation 5:93–102
5. Smith JAR, Norman JN (1982) The fluid of choice for resuscitation of severe shock. Br J Surg 69:702–705
6. Klotz U, Kroemer H (1987) Clinical pharmacokinetic considerations in the use of plasma expanders. Clinical Pharmacokinetics 12:123–135
7. Maningas PA, Mattox KL, Pepe PE, Jones RL, Feliciano DV, Burch JM (1989) Hypertonic saline-dextran solutions for the prehospital management of traumatic hypotension. Am J Surg 157:528–534
8. Kramer GC, Perron PR, Lindsey DC, Ho HS, Gunter RA, et al. (1986) Small-volume resuscitation with hypertonic saline dextran solution. Surgery 100:239–247
9. Brown JM, Grosso MA, Moore EE (1990) Hypertonic saline and dextran: Impact on cardiac function in the isolated rat heart. J Trauma 30:646–651
10. Younes RN, Aun F, Accioly CQ, Casale LP, Szajnbok I, Birolini D (1992) Hypertonic solutions in the treatment of hypovolemic shock: a prospective, randomized study in patients admitted to the emergency room. Surgery 111:380–385
11. McDaniel LB, Nguyen T, Zwischenberger JB, Vertrees R, Uchida T, Kramer GC (1994) Hypertonic saline dextran prime reduces increased intracranial pressure during cardipulmonary bypass in pigs. Anesth Analg 78:435–41
12. Audibert G, Donner M, Lefèvre JC, Stoltz JF, Laxenaire MC (1994) Rheologic effects of plasma substitutes used for preoperative hemodilution. Anesth Analg 78:740–745
13. Funk W, Baldinger V (1995) Microcirculatory perfusion during volume therapy. A comparative study using crystalloid or colloid in awake animals. Anesthesiology 82:975–982

14. Baldwin AL, Wu NZ, Stein AL (1991) Endothelial surface charge of intestinal mucosal capillaries and its modulation by dextran. Microvasc Res 42:160–178
15. Gruber UF, Saldeen T, Brokop T, Eklöf B, Eriksson I et al. (1980) Incidences of fatal postoperative pulmonary embolism after prophylaxis with dextran 70 and low-dose heparin: an international multicentre study. Br Med J i:69–72
16. Nilsson K, Söderlund G (1978) Clinical dextrans. Specifications and quality of preparations on the market. Acta Pharmaceutica Suecica 15:439–454
17. Webb AR, Barclay SA, Bennett ED (1989) In vitro colloid osmotic pressure of commonly used plasma expanders and substitutes: a study of the diffusibility of colloid molecules. Int Care Med 15:116–120
18. Twigley AJ, Hillman KM (1985) The end of the crystalloid era? Anaesthesia 40:860–871
19. Aberg M, Hedner U, Bergentz SE (1979) Effect of dextran on factor VIII (antihaemophilic factor) and platelet function. Ann Surg 189:243–247
20. Ljungström KG (1988) The antithrombotic efficacy of dextran. Acta Chir Scand. Suppl 543:26–30
21. Bergqvist D (1982) Dextran and haemostasis. Acta Chir Scand 148:633–640
22. Bergqvist D (1985) The influence of plasma volume expanders on initial haemostasis in the rabbit mesentery. Acta Anaesthesiol Scand 29:607–609
23. Schött U, Sjöstrand U, Thorén T, Berséus O (1985) Three per cent Dextran-60 as a plasma substitute in blood component therapy. I. An alternative in surgical blood loss replacement. Acta Anaesthesiol Scand 29:767–774
24. Richter AW, Hedin HI (1982) Dextran hypersensitivity. Immunology Today 3:132–138
25. Ljungström KG, Renck H, Strandberg K, Hedin HI, Richter W, Widerlöw E (1983) Adverse reactions to dextran in Sweden 1970–1979 Acta Chir Scand 149:253–262
26. Ljungström KG, Renck H, Hedin H, Richter W, Rosberg B (1983) Prevention of dextran-induced anaphylactic reactions by hapten inhibition. Acta Chir Scand 149:341–348
27. Ljungström KG (1995) Hapten inhibition of dextran reactions. Ten years experience with dextran 1. Br J Anaesth 74:127
28. Perret C, Bedock B, Boles JM, Bussel A, Laxenaire MC, Paillard M, Petit P, Schlemmer B (1989) Choix des produits de remplissage vasculaire pour le traitement des hypovolémies chez l'adulte. IVe Conférence de consensus en réanimation et en médecine d'urgence. Réan Soins intens Méd Urg 5:295–304

CHAPTER 5

Volume Replacement in the Critically Ill   5

J. BOLDT

Introduction

Effective fluid therapy is a mainstay of managing the critically ill patient. Vigorous fluid replacement improves venous return, cardiac output and tissue perfusion. During (hypovolemic-related) low output syndrome (LOS) the body tries to compensate perfusion deficits by redistribution of flow to vital organs (e.g. heart and brain) resulting in an underperfusion of splanchnic bed, kidney, muscles, and skin. Various inflammatory mediators and circulating vasoactive substances are of particular importance for deteriorated perfusion in this situation. Activation of the sympathetic nervous system is one of the compensatory mechanisms to maintain peripheral perfusion. Although this compensatory neurohumoral activation is beneficial at first, this mechanism becomes deleterious and may be involved in the poor outcome of the critically ill. Thus volume therapy should not also tend to optimize macrocirculation and oxygen delivery but also to improve microcirculation. There have been several approaches to defining the optimal type of volume replacement in the critically ill (Table 5.1).

Alternatives to Volume Therapy with Albumin

Albumin is tremendously expensive and acceptable alternatives are urgently needed. Because of cost containment strategies, synthetic colloids are being increasingly used for volume replacement even in the critically ill patient. Gelatin is available in two major

Table 5.1. Important aspects of an ideal volume therapy

Hemodynamic efficacy
Improvement of microcirculation
Beneficial influence on interstitial fluid
No alterations of coagulation
Fewer side effects
Availability
No accumulation
Cost

modifications, modified fluid gelatin and urea-bridged gelatin, the only major differences consisting of different electrolyte concentrations. The increase in blood volume is approximately the same as that of the infused volume of gelatin (range 70%–90%). However, due to the low molecular weight average (approximately 35,000), the plasma half-life is short (1–2 h) so that re-infusions are necessary to maintain blood volume sufficiently. The high incidence of anaphylactic reactions mediated by histamine liberation has been lowered by reducing the amount of cross-linked agents and no longer appears to be a significant problem.

Hydroxyethylstarch solution (HES) is becoming more and more commonly used for volume therapy and fluid replacement in many centres. However, there are several kinds of HES preparations available, which differ with regard to their concentrations (3%, 6%, 10%), degree of substitution (DS) (0.5; 0.62; 0.7), and molecular weight (MW) averages (40,000 daltons; 200,000 daltons; 450,000 daltons).

Is There an Ideal Solution for Volume Replacement?

The controversy concerning the ideal kind of volume replacement does not only include the crystalloid/colloid debate but also the colloid/colloid debate [1]. Although there seems to be no convincing clinical advantage to either solution, human albumin is still widely used in several centres and it is considered the gold standard of volume replacement [2, 3]. There is convincing evidence, however, that the use of albumin is associated with possible negative effects. Addition of albumin in severely traumatized patients was shown to result in a higher incidence of pulmonary failure than observed in patients without albumin infusion. This is most likely due to increased leaking into the interstitial space [4]. By contrast, it has been reported that in sepsis HES may have occlusive effects on damaged capillaries thus limiting extravasation of fluid. Low molecular-weight HES (LMW-HES) may have beneficial effects on endothelial function, e.g. by alteration of endothelial cell integrity in response to O_2 free radical scavenging [6] or by stabilization of fragile cell membranes [7]. This may be of benefit particularly in patients suffering from endothelial leakage syndrome.

Restoration of flow is essential for avoiding tissue ischemia and subsequent development of multiple organ failure (MOF) [8, 9]. However, which solution is best for avoiding the sequelae of trauma or sepsis remains controversial. In a study of ICU (trauma and sepsis) patients the effects of long-term infusion (over 5 days) exclusively with either albumin 20% or 10% HES 200,000/0.5 on important regulators of macro- and microcirculation were investigated [10]. In trauma patients, concentrations of important regulators of circulation showed an almost similar course in both groups. In both sepsis groups, however, plasma levels of vasopressors (vasopressin, endothelin-1, norepinephrine and epinephrine) were significantly elevated. Within the investigation period vasopressor levels decreased significantly, with a more pronounced decline in the HES- than in the albumin-treated patients. Atrial natriuretic peptide (ANP) increased in the albumin patients, 6-keto-prostaglandin F_{1a} (the stable but inactive end product of prostaglandin I_2 [prostacyclin]) plasma levels decreased significantly only in the HES-treated sepsis patients. Summarizing the results it can be assumed that volume replacement with albumin and HES in trauma patients results in similar plasma levels of important regulators of macro- and microcirculation. In sepsis patients, plasma levels of these regulators are more beneficially modified by volume replacement with HES than by albumin infusion. Although macrocirculation did not differ significantly in this study, this may result in beneficial effects on tissue organ perfusion.

In a recent study, critically ill patients received either 500 ml of gelatin or high-molecular weight HES (HMW-HES; average molecular weight 450,000 daltons) and the patients were extensively monitored for 30 min [11]. Although no significant differences in cardiorespiratory effects were seen, the authors concluded from their data that in particular patients (e.g. ARDS-patients) modified fluid gelatin may have an advantage over HMW-HES. Unfortunately, any cardiorespiratory data were acquired after the 30 min-long investigation period. This appears to be extremely important because of the low hemodynamic half-life of gelatin.

Critical illness is often associated with an acute inflammatory response. A complex network of cellular and humoral defense mechanisms are involved in the repair and healing processes. During inflammation, endothelial-derived adhesion molecules are upregulated on the endothelial surface to act with circulating (activated) leukocytes. Tumor necrosis factor (TNF-α) and interleukin (IL)-1 are cytokines which synergistically induce up-regulation of adhesion molecules, thus promoting leukocyte adherence to the endothelium and inducing or maintaining the inflammatory process. Soluble forms of these adhesion molecules have been detected in circulating blood under various conditions and may serve as markers of endothelial activation and damage. In a randomized study, 42 patients with sepsis secondary to major surgery received exclusively either LMW-HES (mean molecular weight 200,000 daltons, DS 0.5) or human albumin for volume therapy over 5 days after diagnosis of sepsis [12]. From arterial blood samples, plasma levels of soluble adhesion molecules (endothelial leukocyte adhesion molecule-1 [soluble ELAM-1], intercellular adhesion molecule-1 [soluble ICAM-1], vascular cell adhesion molecule-1 [soluble VCAM-1], and soluble granule membrane protein 140 [soluble GMP-140] were serially measured. Volume therapy with human albumin failed to beneficially influence plasma levels of adhesion molecules, whereas volume replacement with HES resulted in a decrease in plasma levels of all measured adhesion molecules. The reasons for this can only be speculated on at the moment. Leukocyte adhesion and subsequent endothelial activation are most pronounced in the venular network because shear rates in the venules are rather low. The forces promoting leukocyte/endothelial adhesion and the hemodynamic dispersal forces counteracting it are normally balanced. Macro- and microcirculation are known to be markedly improved by HES [13] resulting either in less expression or less release of adhesion molecules into the circulating blood. Infusion of human albumin did not have this beneficial effect on microperfusion.

Risks of Fluid Therapy

Documented and theoretical hazards are associated with all fluids used for volume therapy. The particular concerns regarding the use of HES include possible alterations in the coagulation system, severe anaphylactic reactions, and development of renal failure [14].

The mechanisms by which synthetic colloids induce coagulation abnormalities (e.g. platelet dysfunction) have not been fully elucidated. In a study of 20 patients with severe sepsis and systemic hypoperfusion, the effects of approximately 1,000 ml of LMW-HES on coagulation were not significantly different than those seen following infusion of the same amount of 5% human serum albumin [15].

HMW-HES diminished the concentrations of VIIIR:Ag and VIIIR:RCo more pronouncedly than did LMW-HES. After large doses of HMW-HES, platelets appeared swollen and platelet adhesion was reduced. Medium or low molecular weight HES (MW 200,000 daltons; MW 70,000 daltons) was reported to have overall fewer negative effects on the coagulation system [15, 16]. In a study of cardiac surgery patients, it was shown that HMW-HES (450,000/0.7) resulted in the overall most pronounced impairment of platelet aggregation and should be avoided in patients with an increased risk of higher postoperative bleeding [17]. LMW-HES did not show the same negative effects on platelet aggregation as were seen in the HMW-HES group. Thus low or medium molecular weight HES (70,000 or 200,000 daltons) and a low DS (0.5) is recommended for volume therapy in patients with risk of bleeding.

In a prospective randomized study of 300 critically ill traumatized (n=150) and septic (n=150) patients, the effects of volume replacement with HES 200/0.5 over 5 days on hemodynamics, laboratory data, and organ function were compared with volume therapy using exclusively human albumin [18]. Mortality during and after the study did not differ significantly between the infusion groups. There were also no differences between the incidence of pulmonary, renal or hepatic failure in the two subgroups. MAP, heart rate (HR), and PCWP were similar in both subgroups, whereas cardiac index (CI), DO_2I, VO_2I, and PaO_2/FIO_2 were higher in the HES- than in the albumin-treated groups. Standard coagulation parameters did not differ, albumin concentration increased significantly in the albumin patients, lactate concentration decreased only in the HES sepsis group (from 2.8±0.5 to 1.5±0.4 mg/dl). The volume regime using albumin was significantly more costly than therapy with HES. It was concluded that volume therapy with HES 200/0.5 for 5 days did not show any disadvantages compared with an infusion regime using albumin. Volume replacement using HES 200/0.5 may even be associated with improved hemodynamics. HES 200/05 appears to be a valuable and significantly cheaper alternative to albumin – even for prolonged and repetitive volume therapy in the critically ill.

Conclusions

In spite of an immense number of studies and proposals regarding the best volume replacement strategy in the critically ill patient, there is still no ideal solution. Whether the choice of fluid does have an impact on patient's outcome is not definitely clear. There seems to be no convincing clinical advantage with respect to patients' outcome with either solution. However, most studies only compared short-term effects of volume infusion (e.g. [19]), and complete assessment of the efficacy of the various volume replacement regimes in the critically ill is not possible with this type of study design. Nevertheless, fluid therapy cannot be the only factor influencing outcome in the critically ill patient. The lack of acceptance of HES for volume replacement is most likely due to reports of abnormal coagulation function [14]. This can no longer be used as an argument against HES because new HES preparations with a low molecular weight (70,000 or 200,000 dalton) and a low DS (0.5) do not negatively influence coagulation.

References

1. Edwards JD (1994) A new debate: colloid versus colloid? In: Vincent JL (ed): Yearbook of intensive care and emergency medicine. Springer, Berlin Heidelberg New York pp 152–164
2. Gressier M, Lehot JJ, George M, Dupraz F, Bastien O, Estanove S (1994) Albumin use and abuse after cardiac surgery. J Cardiothorac Vasc Anesth (suppl 3) 82
3. Kapila A, Waldman CS, Uncles DR, Addy EV (1995) Survey of colloid usage in British intensive care units. Clin Intensive Care 6:A201
4. Weaver DW, Ledgerwood AM, Lucas CE, Higgins R, Bouwman DL, Johnson SD (1978) Pulmonary effects of albumin resuscitation for severe hypovolemic shock. Arch Surg 113:387–39
5. Webb AR, Barclay SA, Bennett ED (1989) In vitro colloid osmotic pressure of commonly used plasma substitutes: A study of the diffusibility of colloid molecules. Intensive Care Med 15:116–120
6. van der Heide RS, Sobotka PA, Gronte CE (1987) Effects of the free radical scavenger DMTU and mannitol on the oxygen paradox in perfused rat hearts. J Mol Cell Cardiol 19:619
7. Justics AC, Farnsworth WV, Soberman MS (1991) Reduction of myocardial infarct size by poloxamer 188 and mannitol in canine model. Am Heart J 122:671
8. Lewis DH (1988) The effects of multiple organ failure on the regulation of the circulation with special reference to the microcirculation. In: Manabe H, Zweifach BW, Messmer K (eds) Microcirculation in circulatory disorders. Springer, Tokyo Berlin Heidelberg, pp 103–108
9. Kirkpatrik CJ, Klosterhalfen B, Hauptmann S (1992) The role of the endothelium in multiple organ failure. In: Vincent JL (ed) Yearbook of intensive care and emergency medicine. Springer, Berlin Heidelberg New York, pp 14–24
10. Boldt J, Müller M, Mentges D, Papsdorf M, Hempelmann G (1996) Influence of different volume therapy regime on regulators of circulation in the critically ill. Br J Anaesth 77:480–487
11. Beards SC, Watt T, Edwards JD, Nightingale P, Farragher EB (1994) Comparison of the hemodynamic and oxygen transport responses to modified fluid gelatin and hetastarch in critically ill patients: a prospective, randomized trial. Crit Care Med 22:600–605
12. Boldt J, Müller M, Heesen M, Martin K, Hempelmann G (1996) Influence of different volume therapies and pentoxifylline infusion on circulating

soluble adhesion molecules in critically ill patients. Crit Care Med 24:385–391

13. Boldt J, Zickmann B, Rapin J, Hammermann H, Dapper F, Hempelmann G (1994) Influence of volume replacement with different HES-solutions on microcirculatory blood flow in cardiac surgery. Acta Anaesthesiol Scand 38:432–438

14. Warren BB, Durieux ME (1996) Hydroxyethylstarch: safe or not? Anesth Analg 84:206–212

15. Strauss RG (1981) Review of the effects of hydroxyethyl starch on the blood coagulation system. Transfusion 21:299–309

16. Treib J, Haass A, Pindur G, Grauer MT, Wenzel E, Schimrigk K (1996) All medium starches are not the same: influence of hydroxyethyl substitution of hydroxyethhyl starch on plasma volume, hemorrheologic conditions, and coagulation. Transfusion 36:450–455

17. Boldt J, Knothe Ch, Zickmann B, Andres P, Dapper F, Hempelmann G (1993) Influence of different intravascular volume therapy on platelet function in patients undergoing cardiopulmonary bypass. Anesth Analg 76:1185–1190

18. Boldt J, Müller M, Mentges D, Papsdorf M, Hempelmann G (1998) Volume therapy in the critically ill: is there a difference? Intensive Care Med 24:28–36

19. Edwards JD, Nightingale P, Wilkins RG, Faragher EB (1988) Hemo-dynamic and oxygen transport response to modified fluid gelatin in the critically ill patients. Crit Care Med 17:996–998

CHAPTER 6

Bleeding Complications and Hydroxyethyl Starch: Strategies of Prevention

6

J. TREIB, M. STOLL

Introduction

Hydroxyethyl starch (HES) is often used as plasma substitute for therapy of hypovolemia after trauma, burns, infections or during surgery (London et al. 1989, Shoemaker et al. 1990). As plasma substitute it has been shown to be as effective as albumin (Rackow et al. 1989, Camu et al. 1995), as long as the patient's plasma protein concentration does not drop below critical levels (Hankeln et al. 1990). Important advantages of HES are the absence of a risk of infection, the low risk of anaphylactic reactions and the low price. HES is also widely used for hemodilution treatment in cerebral (The Hemodilution in Stroke Study Group 1989, Koller et al. 1990, Haass et al. 1992, Stoll et al. 1998), retinal (Arend et al. 1991) and otogenic (Zennaro et al. 1993) perfusion disturbances and in peripheral artery occlusive disease (Kiesewetter et al. 1987). Other indications are hyperdynamic treatment of vasospasm in subarachnoid hemorrhage (Mori et al. 1995) and placenta insufficiency (Molendijk et al. 1995, Bsteh et al. 1995). Some of these indications require high dosages of HES to ensure efficacy of therapy.

Nonetheless, in the past, there have been some reports of bleeding complications during high dose therapy with HES (Symington 1986, Bianchine 1987, Cully et al. 1987, Damon et al. 1987, Sanfelippo et al. 1987, Abramson 1988, Lockwood et al. 1988, Chang et al. 1990, Penner et al. 1990, Dalrymple et al., Lazarchick et al. 1995). Even recently Trumble et al. (1995) reported bleeding complications during hydroxyethyl starch therapy of vasospasm in subarachnoid hemorrhage. Almost all of bleeding complications involved the use of starch with high mean molecular weight (hetastarch), although van den Brink et al. (1996) observed coagulopathy following therapy with medium molecular weight (MW) HES. These reports led to uncertainty about the therapeutic safety of HES. Trumble et al. (1995) even recommended the use of plasma protein fraction instead.

With this background, we investigated the effects of long-term hemodilution treatment of patients with cerebrovascular disease and tested five different HES preparations (Treib et al. 1995, Treib et al. 1996, Stoll et al. 1998). Beside pharmacokinetics and hemorheology we were particularyl interested in the effects on the coagulation system.

Chemical Structure of Hydroxyethyl Starch

HES is a macromolecule consisting of multiple glucose units, which are linked within the chain by a-1,4-glycoside bonds and at branching points by a-1,6 connections. Hydroxyethylation is possible on the C2, C3 or C6 atom. Figure 6.1 shows a portion of the HES macromolecule. HES is manufactured through hydrolysis and subsequent hydroxyethylation from the highly branched starch compound amylopectin. World-wide, many different HES preparations are used which differ in concentration, medium in vitro molecular weight and degree and pattern of hydroxyethylation. Commonly used concentrations of HES are 10%, 6% or 3%. In all HES preparations the weights of the individual molecules are not uniform but rather polydisperse; values given for the molecular weight are therefore mean values. High MW HES (hetastarch) has a mean molecular weight of about 450,000 daltons, medium MW of about 200,000 daltons and low MW HES less than 100,000 daltons. Hydroxyethylation is described by the degree of substitution and the C2/C6 hydroxyethylation ratio. There are starches with a high degree (0.6–0.7) and a low degree (0.4–0.5) of substitution and a high (>8) or low (<8) C2/C6 ratio. Usually the concentration, the mean in vitro molecular weight, the degree of substitution and the C2/C6 ratio are specified in a HES preparation, for example 6% HES 200/0.5/6.

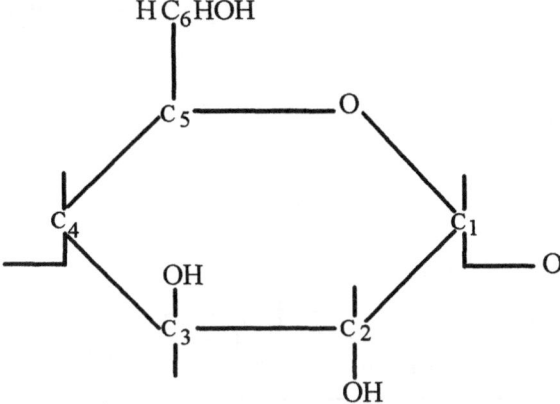

Fig. 6.1. Anhydroglucose-unit with α-1,4- glycosidic bond

Pharmacokinetics of Hydroxyethyl Starch

The chemical structure of HES preparations has important consequences. Polydispersity means that in a HES solution the molecular weight might range from 3000 to 3 million daltons. In vivo, after infusion of a HES solution, molecules smaller than the renal threshold are eliminated by the kidneys, while large molecules are cleaved by α-amylases. The velocity of this cleaving process depends very much on the degree of hydroxyethylation and the hydroxyethylation pattern. Unsubstituted starch is degraded in vivo within minutes by α-amylases. Hydroxyethylation slows down this process and prolongs the effect of starch solutions. The degradation is also slowed by branches in the macromolecule, which are a result of hydroxyethylation at C2. So the rate of enzymatic breakdown can be altered by varying the degree and pattern of hydroxyethylation (Yoshida et al. 1973, Yoshida et al. 1984). Therefore the in vivo mean molecular weight usually differs substantially from the original in vitro mean molecular weight of the HES preparation and is not only predicted by the original in vitro mean molecular weight, but also by the degree of hydroxyethylation and the hydroxyethylation pattern. In our investigations of five different HES solutions (Treib et al. 1995, Treib et al. 1996) 10% HES 200/0.62/10 showed the slowest degradation rate, be-

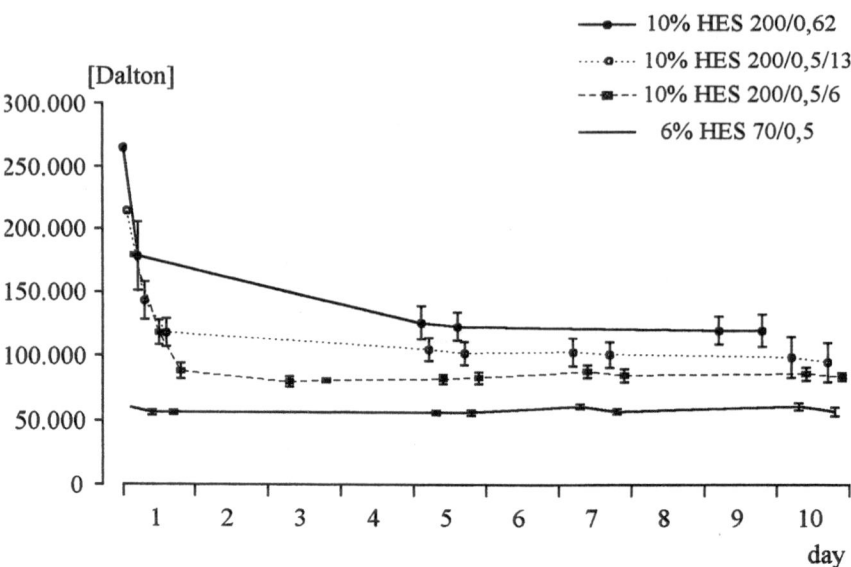

Fig. 6.2. Hydroxyethyl starch (HES) molecular weight during a 10-day volume therapy

cause it has a high degree of substitution and a high C2/C6 ratio (Fig. 6.2). The small molecules of the solution were rapidly eliminated by the kidneys, while the molecules above the renal threshold were only slowly degraded and accumulated (Fig. 6.3). So the mean in vivo molecular weight of 120,000 daltons was much higher than in comparable solutions and the serum concentration increased up to 25.3 g/l. Of the investigated medium MW HES solutions HES 200/0.5/6 had the lowest degree of substitution and the lowest C2/C6 ratio. This led to the lowest mean molecular weight in vivo, only slightly higher than that of low MW HES, and no accumulation, even after 10 days therapy, as the values for HES serum concentration indicated. Low MW HES 70/0.5/4 (also called HES 40/0.5) hardly changes its initial molecular weight (60,000 daltons) in vivo. This starch shows no increase in serum concentration because there are no macromolecules that are difficult to degrade and which can accumulate.

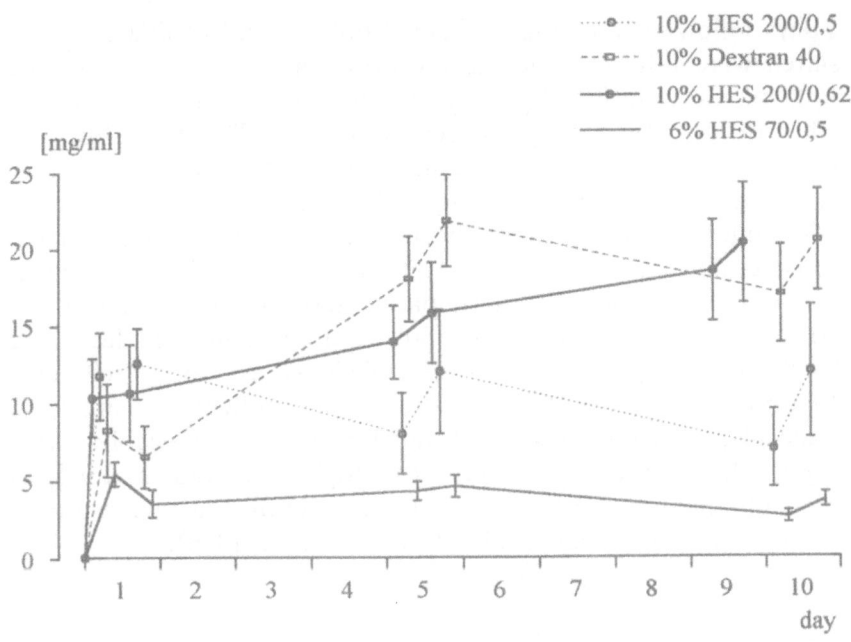

Fig. 6.3. Hydroxyethyl starch (HES) and dextran serum concentration during a 10-day volume therapy

Effects of Hydroxyethyl Starch on Rheology

The pharmacokinetic characteristics of the different HES preparations have a decisive influence on the rheological parameters hematocrit, plasma viscosity and erythrocyte aggregation. Hematocrit changes depend mainly on the volume effect, which is influenced by the HES concentration and the oncotic effect. The 10% solutions of HES 200/0.5 have an additional volume binding effect of 50%–100% of the infused volume (Köhler et al. 1982), while a 6% solution of low MW HES has no volume binding capacity (Messmer and Jesch 1978). For this reason 10% solutions of medium MW HES are usually administered together with electrolyte solution, which is not necessary when using 6% HES. Figure 6.4 shows the change of hematocrit in our investigations. According to our studies, 10% HES 200/0.62/10 had the strongest and longest-lasting volume effect, taking into account that during the first

4 days following the „loading dose" only 500 ml of this particular starch were infused, whereas the dose for all other starches was 1000 ml. Considering that only 6% solution was used, the volume effect of low MW starch was relatively large. This underlines that it is not the size of the molecules, but the number of oncotically active molecules that determine the volume effect.

Changes of plasma viscosity and erythrocyte aggregation vary considerably among different HES solutions. A rheologically advantageous decrease of these parameters is only achieved with HES having an in vivo molecular weight of less than 90,000 daltons (Haass et al. 1992, Treib et al. 1995, Treib et al. 1996, Stoll et al. 1998) and is due to the influence of small HES molecules. In contrast, an accumulation of large molecules, which occurs during the administration of high MW HES or slowly degradable medium MW HES, results in a significant increase of the plasma viscosity (Treib et al. 1995, Treib et al. 1996).

Effects of Hydroxyethyl Starch on the Coagulation System

The disturbances of the coagulation system caused by HES were found to be due to an acquired von Willebrand syndrome type I (Stump et al. 1985, Sanfelippo 1987, Dalrymple et al. 1992, Conroy et al. 1996, Treib et al. 1996). The decrease of von Willebrand factor (vWF) VIII is thought to be caused by the accumulation of large HES molecules when using high MW HES. As mentioned above this accumulation can also be found when using slowly degradable medium MW HES, which explains the observation of van den Brink et al. (1996). We were also able to show that medium MW HES, which is highly substituted or has a high C2/C6 ratio, has the same undesired properties as starch with high MW, which explains the bleeding complications reported by van den Brink et al.

In our investigation of five different HES preparations (Treib et al. 1995, Treib et al. 1996, Treib et al. 1997) we also assessed influences on the coagulation system by measuring thromboplastin time (Quick), activated partial thromboplastin time (PTT) and thrombin time (Figs. 6.5, 6.6). In order to evaluate an impairment

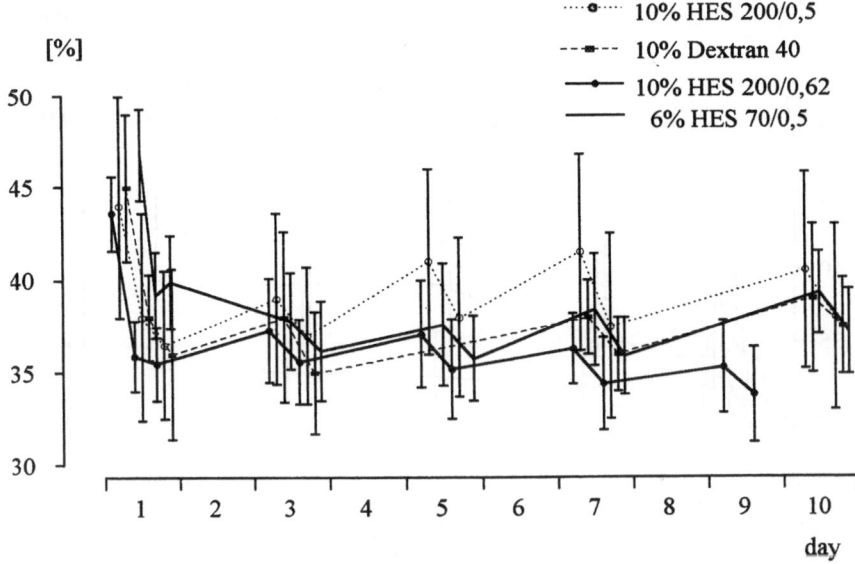

Fig. 6.4. Change of hematocrit during a 10-day volume therapy with hydroxyethyl starch (HES) or dextran

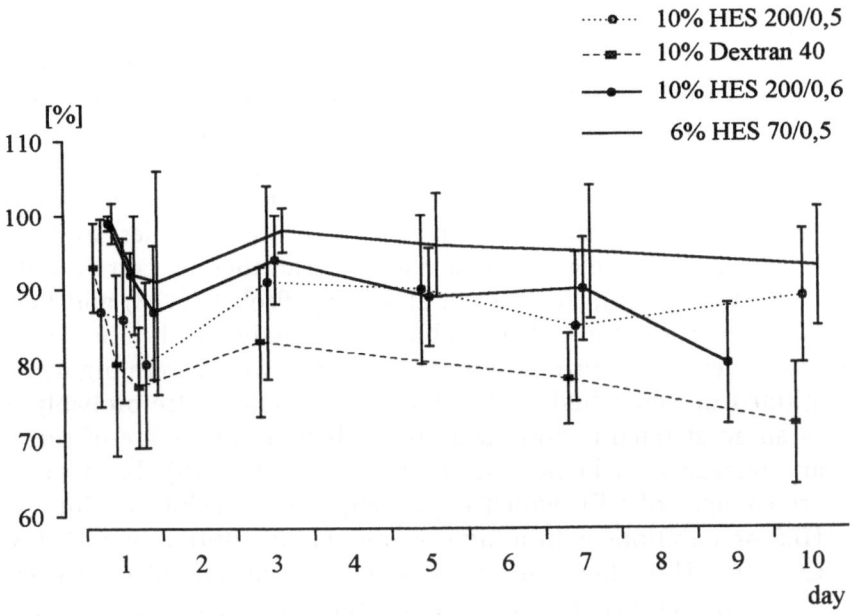

Fig. 6.5. Change of thromboplastin time (Quick) during a 10-day volume therapy

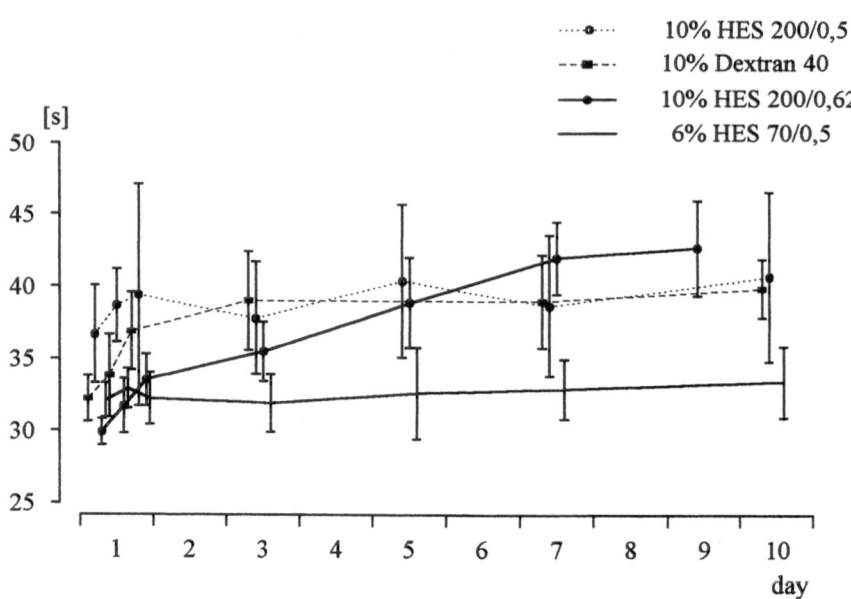

Fig. 6.6. Change of activated partial thromboplastin time (PTT) during a 10-day volume therapy

of vWF VIII we also measured the different vWF VIII subunits: factor VIII:C, von Willebrand ristocetin cofactor and von Willebrand factor antigen (Figs. 6.7–6.9). A relevant reduction of thromboplastin time (Quick) could only be found when using 10% HES 200/0.62/10. The other HES solutions did not change thromboplastin time. These results agree with earlier studies of thromboplastin time during a one-day HES therapy carried out by Peter et al. (1975), Vinazzer et al. (1975), Probst (1988) and Reiger (1988). A shortening of thrombin time together with a decrease of fibrinogen could also be found in starches which were highly substituted or had a high C2/C6 ratio. These effects are probably due to an accelerated polymerization of fibrin and they are of secondary relevance to hemostasis (Vinazzer et al. 1975). Most notable are changes of PTT, which is prolonged when using medium MW HES preparations with a high degree of substitution or a high C2/C6 ratio. This effect on PTT is due to a substantial reduction of vWF VIII activity by these starch preparations. A decrease in factor vWF VIII rarely leads to spontaneous bleedings but may con-

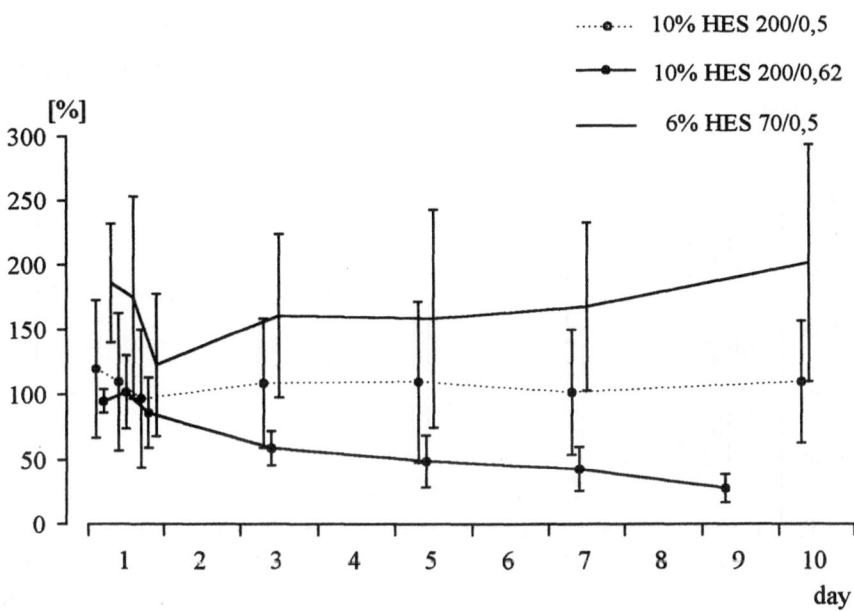

Fig. 6.7. Change of factor VIII:C during a 10-day volume therapy

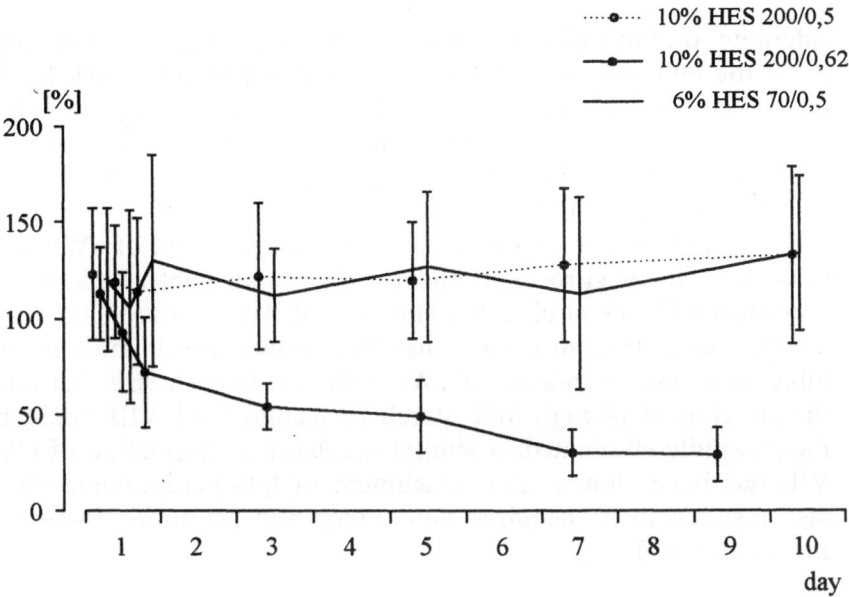

Fig. 6.8. Change of von Willebrand ristocetin cofactor during a 10-day volume therapy

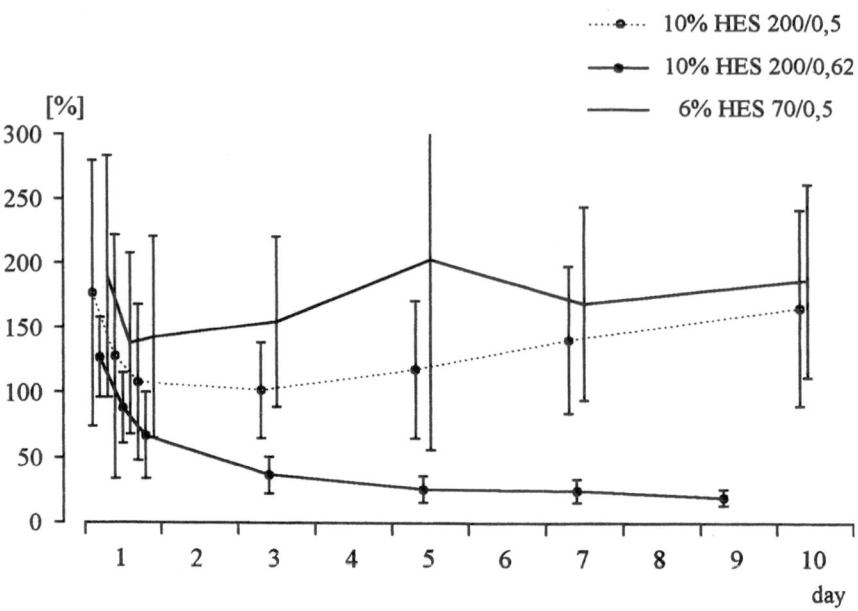

Fig. 6.9. Change of von Willebrand factor antigen during a 10-day volume ther-

siderably prolong bleeding from even small injuries. vWF supports the adhesion of platelets to the injured blood vessel. Medium or low MW HES with a low degree of substitution and a low C2/C6 ratio does not effect vWF activity and PTT beyond the dilution effect, even when high dosages are administered (Treib et al. 1996, Stoll et al. 1998).

So far the precise pathogenesis of the impairment of vWF VIII is unclear. In in vitro experiments this impairment could not be reproduced (Batlle et al. 1985, Stump et al. 1985, Grauer and Treib 1998), and it was suspected that HES either precipitates or inhibits synthesis or release of vWF VIII. We hypothesize that after the attachment of high MW starch molecules vWF VIII might be more rapidly eliminated. A similar accelerated elimination of vWF VIII has been shown after attachment of IgG paraprotein, which also resulted in an acquired von Willebrand syndrome (Siostrzonek et al. 1985).

Conclusions and Consequences for Clinical Use of Hydroxyethyl Starch

Our investigations demonstrate that most of the undesired effects of HES, which are mainly accumulation, impairment of the coagulation system and unfavourable rheologic influences, are caused by HES macromolecules with very high MWs. Because of the polydispersity of HES solutions these macromolecules are a regular part of high or medium MW HES preparations. For elimination the macromolecules have to be cleaved by α-amylases until their molecular size is smaller than the renal threshold. The velocity of this cleaving process depends on the degree of hydroxyethylation and on the share of C2-hydroxyethylated starch molecules. In HES solutions with a high initial MW (for example HES 450/0.7, hetastarch) and in solutions with medium MW and a high degree of hydroxyethylation (for example HES 200/0.62/10) or a high C2/C6 ratio (for example HES 200/0.5/13) the cleaving velocity is too small, which leads to an accumulation of these macromolecules and a high in vivo MW during long-term therapy. By contrast, medium MW HES solutions, which have a low degree of substitution and a low C2/C6 ratio (for example HES 200/0.5/6), or low MW HES solutions (for example HES 70/0.5/4) have a low in vivo MW and show no accumulation of macromolecules. Therefore, hemorrhagic complications and negative rheologic influences can be avoided by choosing an appropriate starch with a low in vivo MW.

References

Abramson N (1988) Plasma Expanders and Bleeding. Ann Intern Med 108:307

Arend O, Hoberg A, Bertram B, Reim M, Wolf S (1991) Hemodilution in acute arterial circulatory disorders of the retina. Acta-Med-Austriaca 18 Suppl1:66–68

Batlle J, Del Rio F, Fernandez MF, Martin R, Borrasca A (1985) Effect of dextran on factor VIII/von Willebrand factor structure and function. Thromb Haemostas 54:697–9

Bianchine JR (1987) To the editor. N Engl J Med 317:965

van den Brink WA, van Genderen P, Thijsse WJ, Michiels JJ (1996) Hetastarch Coagulopathy. J Neurosurg 85:367

Bsteh M, Tews G, John D (1995) Hämodilution bei der Behandlung der intrauterinen Dystrophie. Geburtsh Frauenheilk 55:83–86

Camu F, Ivens D, Christiaens F (1995) Human albumine and colloid fluid replacement: their use in general surgery. Acta Anaesthesiol Belg 46:3–18

Chang JC, Gross HM, Jang NS (1990) Disseminated intravascular coagulation due to intravenous administration of hetastarch. Am J Med Sci 300:301–303

Conroy JM, Fishman RL, Reeves ST, Pinosky ML, Lazzarchick J (1996) The effect of desmopressin and 6% hydroxyethyl starch on factor VIII:C. Anaesth Analg 83:804–807

Cully MD, Larson CP, Silverberg GD (1987) Hetastarch coagulopathy in a neurosurgical patient. Anaesthesiology 66:707–708

Dalrymple HM, Aitchison R, Collins P, Sekhar M, Colvin B (1992) Hydroxyethyl starch induced acquired von Willebrand~Os disease. Clin Lab Haematol 14:209–211

Damon L, Adams M, Stricker RB, Ries C (1987) Intracranial bleeding during treatment with hydroxyethyl starch. N Engl J Med 317:964–965

Grauer MT, Treib J. The effect of hydroxyethyl starch on coagulation is diffucult to assess in vitro. Br J Anaesth, in press

Haass A, Stoll M, Treib J (1992) Hemodilution in cerebral circulatory disturbances: indications, implementation additional drug treatment and alternatives. In: Hemodilution. New aspects in the management of circulatory blood flow. Improvement of macro- and microcirculation. Springer Berlin Heidelberg New York p 53–114

Haass A, Treib J, Stoll M (1992) Hemorheological parameters of hydroxyethyl starch 200/0.62 as a basis for hemodilution. Clin Hemorheol 12:17–26

Hankeln K, Senker R, Beez M (1990) Comparative study of the intraoperative efficacy of 5% human albumin and 10% hydroxyethyl starch (HES-steril) in terms of hemodynamics and oxygen transport in 40 patients. Infusionsther Transfusionsmed 17:135–140

Hemodilution in Stroke Study Group (1989) Hypervolemic hemodilution treatment of acute stroke. Results of a randomized multicenter trial using pentastarch. Stroke 20:317–323

Kiesewetter H, Jung F, Blume J, Gerhards M (1987) Hämodilution bei Patienten mit peripherer arterieller Verschlußkrankheit im Stadium IIb: Prospektiver randomisierter Doppelblind-Vergleich von mittelmolekularer Hydroxyethylstärke und kleinmolekularer Dextranlösung. Klin Wschr 65:324–330

Köhler H, Zschiedrich H, Clasen R, Linfante A, Gamm H (1982) Blutvolumen, kolloidosmotischer Druck und Nierenfunktion von Probanden nach Infusion von mittelmolekularer 10% Hydroxyäthylstärke 200/0,5 und 10% Dextran 40. Anaesthesist 31:61–67

Koller M, Haenny P, Hess K, Weniger D, Zangger P (1990) Adjusted hypervolemic hemodilution in acute ischemic stroke. Stroke 21:1429–1434

Lazarchick J, Conroy JM (1995) The effect of 6% hydroxyethyl starch and desmopressin infusion on von Willebrand factor: ristocetin cofactor activity. Ann Clin Lab Sci 25:306–309

Lockwood DNJ, Bullen C, Machin SJ (1988) A severe coagulophathy following volume replacement with hydroxyethylstarch in a jehovah's witness. Anaesthesia 43:391–393

London MJ, Ho Js, Triedman JK, Verrier ED, Levine J, Merrick SH, Hanley FL, Browner WS, Mangono DT (1989) A randomized clinical trial of 10% pentastarch (low molecular weight hydroxyethyl starch) versus 5% albumin for plasma volume expansion after cardiac operations. J Thorac Cardiovasc Surg 97:785–797

Messmer K, Jesch F (1978) Volumenersatz und Hämodilution durch Hydroxyäthylstärke. Infusionstherapie 5:169–177

Molendijk L, Malburg I, Kopecky P (1995) Dopplersonographische Untersuchungen bei Plazentainsuffizienz als Hinweis auf die Effektivität der Hämodilutionstherapie. Z Geburtshilfe Perinatol 199:18–22

Mori K, Arai H, Nakajima K, Tajima A, Maeda M (1995) Hemorheological and hemo dynamic analysis of hypervolemic hemodilution therapy for cerebral vasospasm after aneurysmal subarachnoid hemorrhage. Stroke 26:1620–1626

Penner M, Fingerhut D, Tacke A (1990) Effect of a new 10% hydroxyethyl starch solution HES/270/0.5 on blood coagulation, blood loss and hemodynamics in comparison with 3.5% PPL. Infusionstherapie 17:314–318

Peter K, Gander HP, Lutz H, Nold W, Strosiek U (1975) Die Beeinflussung der Blutgerinnung durch Hydroxyäthylstärke. Anaesthesist 24:219–224

Probst W (1988) Elohäst (Hydroxyethylstärke 6% 200/0.60–0.66) bei akuten ischämischen cerebralen Durchblutungsstörungen. Elohäst Workshop 11–12

Rackow EC, Mecher C, Astiz ME, Griffel M, Falk JL, Weil MH (1989) Effects of pentastarch and albumin infusion on cardiorespiratory function and cogulation in patients with severe sepsis and systemic hypoperfusion. Crit Care Med 17:394–398

Reiger I (1988) Erfahrungen mit Elohäst (Hydroxyethylstärke 6% 200/0.60–0.66) in der Therapie des Cerebralinsults. Elohäst Workshop 10

Sanfelippo MJ, Suberviola PD, Geimer NF (1987) Development of a von Willebrand like syndrom after prolonged use of hydroxyethyl starch. Am J Clin Pathol 88:653–655

Shoemaker WC, Kram HB (1990) Effects of crystalloids and colloids on hemodynamics, oxygen transport and outcome in high-risk surgical patients. In: Simmons RC, Udekuo AS (eds.). Debates in clinical surgery. Yearbook, Chicago 263–316

Siostrzonek P, Niessner H, Deutsch E, Lechner K, Korninger C, Pabinger I, Heinz R (1985) Vier Fälle mit erworbenem von Willebrand-Syndrom und monoklonaler Gammopathie. Langzeitverlauf sowie diagnostische und therapeutische Problematik. In: 16. Hämophilie Symposion, Hamburg. Landbeck G, ed. Springer, Berlin – Heidelberg – New York, pp 248–56

Stoll M, Treib J, Schenk F, Windisch F, Haass A, Wenzel E, Schimrigk K (1998) No coagulation disorders under high dose volume therapy with low molecular weight hydroxyethyl starch. Haemostasis, in press

Stoll M, Treib J, Seltmann A, Haass A, Schimrigk K (1998) Hemodynamics of stroke patients under therapy with low molecular weight hydroxyethyl starch. Neurol Res (in press)

Stump DC, Strauss RG, Henriksen RA, Petersen RE, Saunders R (1985) Effects of hydroxyethyl starch on blood coagulation, particularly factor VIII. Transfusion 25:349–354

Symington BE (1986) Hetastarch and bleeding complications. Ann Intern Med 105:627–628

Treib J, Haaß A, Pindur G, Seyfert UT, Treib W, Grauer MT, Jung F, Wenzel E, Schimrigk K (1995) HES 200/0,5 is not HES 200/0,5. Influence of the C2/C6 hydroxyethylation ratio of hydroxyethyl starch (HES) on hemorheology, coagulation and elimination kinetics. Thromb Haemost 74:1452–1456

Treib J, Haaß A, Pindur G, Grauer MT, Wenzel E, Schimrigk K (1996) Abnahme des Thrombozytenvolumens durch mehrtägige Infusion von hochsubstituierter mittelmolekularer Hydroxyäthylstärke (HÄS 200/0,62). Wien Klin Wochenschr 108:20–23

Treib J, Haaß A, Pindur G, Treib W, Wenzel E, Schimrigk K (1996) Influence on intravascular molecular weight of hydroxyethyl starch on platelets during a long-term hemodilution. Eur J Hematol 56:168–172

Treib J, Haaß A, Pindur G, Grauer MT, Wenzel E, Schimrigk K (1996) Decrease of fibronectin following repeated infusion of highly substituted hydroxyethyl starch. Infusionsther Transfusionsmed 23:71–75

Treib J, Haaß A, Pindur G, Grauer MT, Wenzel E, Schimrigk K (1996) All medium starches are not the same: Influence of degree of substitution of hydroxyethyl starch on volumen effect, hemorheologic conditions and coagulation. Transfusion 36:450–455

Treib J, Haaß A, Pindur G, Miyachita C, Grauer MT, Jung F, Wenzel E, Schimrigk K (1996) Highly substituted hydroxyethyl starch (HES 200/0.62) leads to a type I von Willebrand syndrome after repeated administration. Haemostasis 26:210–213

Treib J, Haaß A, Pindur G (1996) Hetastarch coagulopathy. J Neurosurg 85:367–368

Treib J, Haaß A, Pindur G, Grauer MT, Seyfert UT, Treib W, Wenzel E, Schimrigk K (1996) Influence of low molecular weight hydroxyethyl starch on hemostasis and hemorheology. Haemostasis 26:258–265

Treib J, Haaß A, Pindur G, Treib W, Wenzel E, Schimrigk K (1996) Influence of low and medium molecular weight hydroxyethyl starch on platelets during a long-term hemodilution. Arzneimittelforschung/Drug Research 46:1064–1066

Treib J, Haaß A (1997) Hydroxyethyl starch. J Neurosurg 86:574–575

Treib J, Haaß A, Pindur G, Grauer MT, Treib W, Wenzel E, Schimrigk K (1997) Increased hemorrhagic risk after repeated infusion of highly substituted medium molecular weight hydroxyethyl starch (10% HES 200/0.62). Arzneimittelforschung/Drug Research 47:18–22

Treib J, Haaß A, Pindur G, Grauer MT, Wenzel E, Schimrigk K (1997) Avoiding an impairment of factor VIII:C by using hydroxyethyl starch with a low in vivo molecular weight. Anesth Analg 84:1391

Treib J, Haaß A, Pindur G, Grauer MT, Wenzel E, Schimrigk K (1997) A more differentiated classification of hydroxyethyl starch is nessessary. Intens Care Med 23:709–710

Treib J, Haaß A, Pindur G (1997) Review article: Coagulation disorders caused by hydroxyethyl starch. Thromb Haemost 78:974–983

Treib J, Haaß A, Pindur G, Wenzel E, Schimrigk K (1997) Blutungskomplikationen durch Hydroxyethylstärke sind vermeidbar. Deutsches Ärzteblatt 94:2326–2330

Treib J, Haaß A, Schimrigk K (1997) European hydroxyethyl starch: a safe and inexpensive alternative to albumine. Anesth Analg 85:709

Treib J, Haaß A (1997) Rheologische Eigenschaften von Hydroxyethylstärke. Dtsch Med Wschr 122:1319–1322

Trumble ER, Muizelaar JP, Myseros JS, Choi SC, Warren BB (1995) Coagulopathy with the use of hetastarch in the treatment of vasospasm. J Neurosurg 82:44–47

Vinazzer H, Bergmann H (1975) Zur Beeinflussung postoperativer Änderungen der Blutgerinnung durch Hydroxyäthylstärke. Anaesthesist 24:517–520

Yoshida M, Yamashita T, Matsuo J, Kishikawa T (1973) Enzymic degradation of hydroxyethyl starch. Part I. Influence of the distribution of hydroxyethyl groups on the enzymic degradation of hydroxyethyl starch. Stärke 25:373–376

Yoshida M, Kishikawa T (1984) A study of hydroxyethyl starch. Part II. Degradation-sites of hydroxyethyl starch by pig pankreas alpha-amylase. Starch/Stärke 36:167–16

Yoshida M, Minami Y, Kishikawa T (1984) A study of hydroxyethyl starch. Part III. Comparison of metabolic fates between 2–0-hydroxyethyl starch and 6–0-hydroxyethyl starch in rabbits. Starch/Stärke 36:209–212

Zennaro O, Dauman R, Poisot A, Esteben D, Duclose JY, Bertrand B, Cros AM, Milacic M, Bebear JP (1993) Value of the association of normovolemic dilution and hyperbaric oxygenation in the treatment of sudden deafness. A retrospective study. Ann-Otolaryngol-Chir-Cervicofac 110:162–169

CHAPTER 7

Volume Replacement in Burn Patients 7

D. BALOGH

Introduction

A severe burn injury is still a life-threatening event. Therefore, it is crucial that every detail of therapy is optimised. One can distinguish different phases in the course of the burn illness: burn shock ($\sim$24 h), ebb and flow phases ($\sim$first week) and the complex syndrome of burn illness (several weeks), which is determined by sequential operations, by the deterioration of various organ systems and by multiple infections. For adequate treatment a knowledge of the complex shift in fluids, proteins and electrolytes is necessary.

Pathophysiology of Burn Injury

A burn injury not only affects the skin, but a cascade of mediators is released from the burned area. These mediators influence capillary permeability and induce plasma and sodium to shift to the interstitial spaces. This exerts a rapid effect on intravascular volume, peripheral tone and microcirculation, resulting in oxygen deficiency of various tissues. A burn injury also causes a dramatic increase in stress hormones affecting metabolism. As result of the high oxygen demand and low oxygen supply, metabolic acidosis develops and further influences cardiac ventricular functions (Fig. 7.1). Burn shock consequently develops, and it caused high mortality before the key role of rapid fluid replacement was recognised [5].

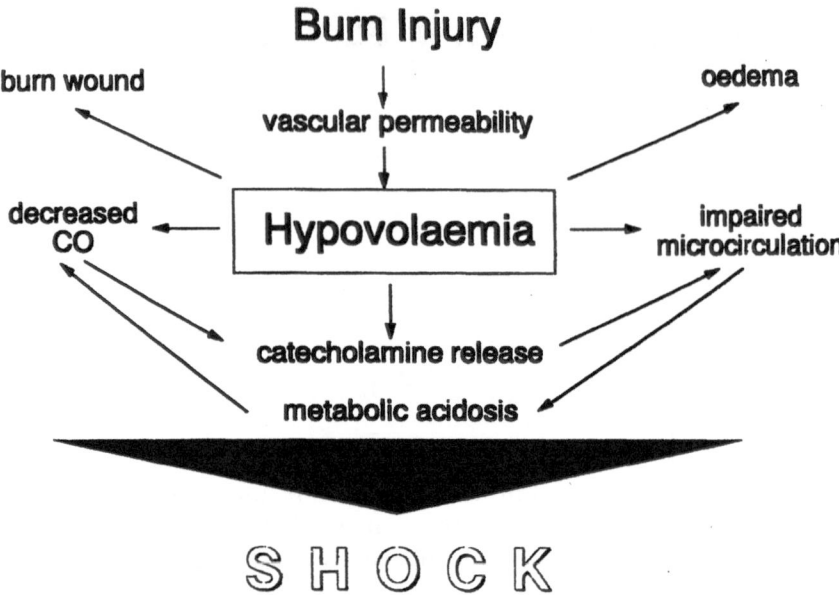

Fig. 7.1. Pathophysiology of burn shock

On admission burn patients show signs of intravascular volume loss: high haematocrit, low plasma sodium with decreased arterial pressure and poor urine excretion; pH values are often in the acidotic range. Fortunately, emergency medicine often starts volume replacement at the site of the accident, so that burn shock will not develop in such a dramatic way.

The extent and duration of capillary leak (ebb phase) depends on the extent of the burn injury, and on whether there is additional trauma, inhalation injury or high-voltage burn. The amount of burn oedema highly depends on the resuscitation regime, i.e. amount and quality of fluid used. Following successful resuscitation, the interstitial oedema will begin to flow back (flow phase) (Fig. 7.2).

In addition to rapid haemodynamic stabilisation, the reduction of burn oedema is a common goal in the resuscitation of thermal injury, so that we can excise and cover third degree burns as early as possible. Transplanted skin can only be expected to take well when there is no substantial interstitial oedema. Burned skin is always prone to bacterial infection, and we should try to excise and

"Ebbe- and Flow-phase"

in burn patients

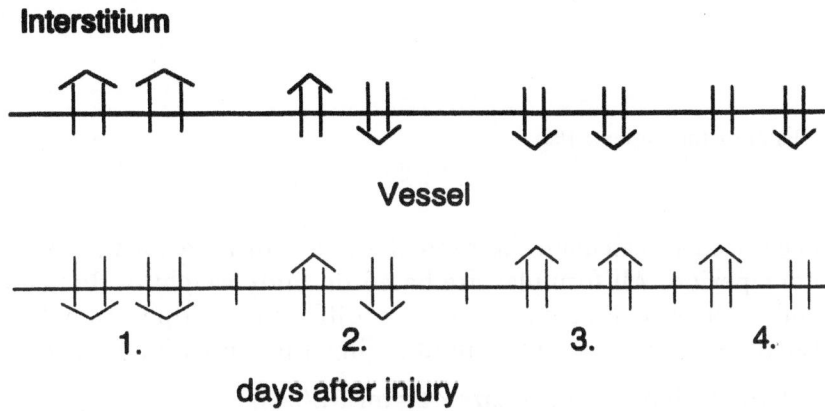

Fig. 7.2. Time course of the ebb and flow phases in burn injury

cover all burns within the first 2 weeks when we can expect the burn wound to still be sterile and no burn wound sepsis to have developed. Interstitial oedema decreases tissue oxygenation, delays healing and can therefore contribute to the development of sepsis syndrome.

Fluid replacement in burns has two different applications: initial fluid resuscitation in burn shock, and fluid replacement of blood and fluid loss during surgery.

Initial Fluid Replacement

There is still no consent on an ideal fluid replacement in burn shock. Such a fluid should guarantee quick restoration of the circulating blood volume while simultaneously minimising oedema formation [1, 3, 6, 11].

Crystalloids as well as colloids have been used to resuscitate burn victims. For the different solutions different formulas have

Table 7.1. Estimation of burned body surface[a] („rule of nine")

	Adults	Children	
		5–10 years	1 year
Head+neck	9	16	20
Trunk	18×2	17×2	17×2
Arms	9×2	9×2	9×2
Legs	18×2	16×2	14×2

[a]Palm of the patient: 1%.

been used to calculate the needed amount of fluid for the first 24-hour period. All formulas are based on body weight of the patient and burn size (Table 7.1) using a different multiplication factor. Currently, the most widely used regimen is the Parkland formula:

Body weight×% burn size×4 = ml RL/24 h

followed by colloids (albumin or plasma) once endothelial competency has been restored. This formula causes an important interstitial oedema. The onset of the flow phase (backflow of oedema), however, starts early, within 36–48 h of injury, so that surgery can start on day 3 after the accident.

Initial fluid resuscitation imports a great amount of sodium (1 l isotonic cristalloid $\simeq$ 140 mmol sodium) that goes mainly into the interstitial oedema and total body sodium increases. During the ebb phase, as soon as the backflow of the interstitial oedema and the interstitial Na^+ commences, we see a steep increase in plasma sodium. Therefore, sodium intake must be strictly reduced after the first 24 h. Pathological plasma sodium levels can develop especially if kidney function is impaired and high sodium excretion in urine is impossible.

All recommended formulas for initial fluid replacement can give only rough guidelines, and it is essential to treat patients according to target values (Table 7.2). Spontaneous urine excretion, haematocrit and colloid osmotic pressure are valuable guidelines for fluid therapy. CVP and PAP are misleading in burn patients, because physiological values can be obtained only by overinfusion, resulting in enormous interstitial oedema.

Table 7.2. Target values

Urine	1 ml/kg per hour
MAP	>60 mm Hg
HR	<120/min
Hk	<50%
COP	>12
Na$^+$	<150 mmol/l
CVP	~5
SvO$_2$	>60%

MAP, mean arterial pressure; HR, heart rate; Hk, haematocrit; COP, colloid osmotic pressure; CVP, central venous pressure; SvO$_2$, mixed venous saturation.

It is clear that many different fluids are effective in restoring hae-modynamics and safeguarding kidney function, but at the cost of tissue oedema and sodium load. It has been proven that hypertonic saline can minimise interstitial oedema while effectively treating burn shock. Various hypertonic solutions have been used up to an osmolarity of 200 mmol Na$^+$/l. Recently, promising results were ob-tained with 7.5% sodium ($\sim$2400 mosmol/l) in combination with an artificial colloid (dextran or hydroxyethyl starch) [9, 10]. Resuscita-tion volume can be reduced but plasma sodium can increase drama-tically, and close monitoring of plasma sodium is necessary to pre-vent a detrimental increase of plasma osmolarity.

Beside hypertonic saline, early application of colloids also re-duces resuscitation volume and tissue oedema. Old historical for-mulas (Muir and Evans) recommended the use of albumin, which should not be used for initial resuscitation because it produces a long-lasting oedema and pulmonary complications [2].

Recently, various studies [4, 8] have compared artificial col-loids, mainly hydroxyethyl starch, with crystalloids and demon-strated a rapid stabilisation of circulation and less tissue oedema. Total sodium intake remained identical for all solutions (isotonic and hypertonic saline, hydroxyethyl starch). The importance of initial sodium input for intravascular volume was confirmed [8, 10]. There is also some evidence to show that large starch mole-cules can alter the microvascular permeability and act as free rad-ical scavengers [4, 8]. Rapid haemodynamic stabilisation in burn shock can be achieved using various solutions once the patho-physiology of burn shock development is understood.

Fluid Replacement for Surgical Interventions

Large burns entail a great number of operations, i.e. excision of burned skin with subsequent coverage. Especially tangential excision causes great blood loss, which is difficult to measure. Good coagulation is crucial for limiting blood loss and for good surgical results. Therefore, in addition to packed red cells, a large amount of fresh frozen plasma is usually needed for fluid replacement and coagulation therapy. As sequential operations are needed for extensive burns, the total amount of fluids used during burn treatment can be very high, exceeding recommended maximum applications for most artificial colloids.

There are some suggestions that chronic use of hydroxyethyl starch could be harmful for burn patients [2, 7, 12]. As tremendous amounts of colloids can be necessary over the long course of burn treatment, all side effects must be weighed carefully. Particularly the storage of hydroxyethyl starch in the reticulo-endothelial system (RES) can be detrimental in immunocompromised patients who are always prone to infection [12].

For temporary replacement of volume loss during surgery gelatin solutions are very useful, because the application is not limited. In addition, as gelatin disintegrates into CO_2 and water, no problems of excretion or long-lasting storage will occur. Allergic reactions are mostly not very severe and can be mitigated by anaesthesia.

Since protein synthesis is diminished in major burns, albumin levels can be low and substitution might be necessary. Albumin can perhaps bind polypeptides, so-called burn toxins, and help in detoxification; low protein levels can also influence the effect of drugs with high protein binding capacity (i.e. benzodiazepam).

Summary

The goal of initial fluid resuscitation in burn patients is circulatory stabilisation with maintenance of vital organ function, with the least immediate or delayed side effects [1, 2, 7, 12]. All efforts should be directed toward minimising oedema formation, so that third degree burned skin can rapidly be excised and covered before bacterial colonisation of the burned skin occurs. For further fluid treatment, the side effects of all solutions must be considered carefully because of a possible cumulative effect.

References

1. Aharoni A (1989) Burn resuscitation with a low-volume plasma regimen – analysis of mortality. Burns 15(4):230–233
2. Aharoni A (1989) Pulmonary complications in burn patients resuscitated with a low-volume colloid solution. Burns 15(5):281–284
3. Bortolani A, Governa M, Barisoni D (1996) Fluid replacement in burned patients. Acta Chir Plast 38:132–136
4. Brazeal BA, Honeycutt D, Traber LD, Toole JG, Herndon DN, Traber DL (1995) Pentafraction for superior resuscitation of the ovine thermal burn. Crit Care Med 23:332–339
5. Carleton SC (1995) Cardiac problems associated with burns. Cardiology Clinics 13:257–262
6. Fakhry SM, Alexander J, Smith D, Meyer AA, Peterson HD (1995) Regional and institutional variation in burn care. J Burn Care Rehabil 16:86–90
7. Gore DC, Dalton JM, Gehr TW (1996) Colloid infusions reduce glomerular filtration in resuscitated burn victims. J Trauma 40:356–360
8. Guha SC, Kinsky MP, Button B, Herndon DN, Traber LD, Traber DL, Kramer GC (1996) Burn resuscitation: crystalloids versus colloids versus hypertonic saline colloid in sheep. Crit Care Med 24:1849–1857
9. Milner SM, Kinsky MP, Herndon DN, Philips IG, Kramer GC (1997) A comparison of two different 2400 mosm solutions for resuscitation of major burns. J Burn Care Rehabil 18:109–115
10. Onarheim H, Missavage AE, Kramer GC, Gunther RA (1990) Effectiveness of hypertonic saline-dextran 70 for initial fluid resuscitation of major burns. J Trauma 30:597–603
11. Shirani KZ, Voughan GM, Mason AD Jr., Pruitt BA Jr (1996) Update on current therapeutic approaches in burns. Shock 5:4–16
12. Trop M, Schiffrin EJ, Callahan R, Carter EA (1992) Effect of heta-starch colloid solutions on reticuloendothelial phagocytic system (RES) function in burned and infected rats. Burns 18:463–465

CHAPTER 8

Use of Plasma Substitutes During Cardiac Surgery: Focus on Priming Solutions

8

D. HIMPE

Introduction

One of the many controversies in the field of cardiopulmonary bypass (CPB) that has not been satisfactorily resolved is the good governance of fluid homeostasis. With the initiation of CPB, an extra void is added to the intravascular space by connecting arterial and venous vascular trees to an ex vivo machinery including plastic tubing, filters, pumps, and an artificial lung. This expansion requires an appropriate solution to fill the extracorporeal circuit. During CPB microvascular permeability can also be affected with an expansion of the interstitial space. This depends on the degree of venous back-pressure, lymphatic circulation, and plasma colloid osmotic pressure (COP). In the early days of cardiac surgery hemodilution was first seen as an undesirable side effect [85]. With the improvement of the oxygenators, the priming volume increased and the use of blood substitutes became unavoidable [27]. Hemodilution soon proved to be effective in preventing the „homologous blood syndrome" and renal problems [15, 70]. Depending on their specific composition, rehydration and replacement solutions can be used for the treatment (restorative or corrective) of different fluid spaces [60]. Although many of these solutions have been used for hemodilution during CPB, there is still no uniformly accepted solution. In 1964, the South Central Association of Blood Banks (USA) already focused on the confusion about the composition of priming solutions [85]. Despite increased knowledge, the confusion has not yet fully disappeared and no consensus has been reached about the most appropriate composition.

Priming Solutions and their Relation to Cardiopulmonary Bypass

Cardiac surgery with CPB can be complicated by a systemic inflammatory response syndrome (SIRS), which has been ascribed to the interfacing of blood with non-endothelial surfaces. Contact activation cascades, the complement system, and cellular elements interact and generate mediators to produce this complex inflammatory response [46]. There may be an interplay between the composition of the priming and these processes [12, 68]. Currently, opinions differ on this subject [74, 90]. In the absence of clear data, charismatic theories are apt to trigger the emergence of dogmatic beliefs. Therefore, many institutions continue to use their own, home-made priming mixes.

Evidence Based Selection of a Priming Solution

This chapter addresses the issue whether the composition of the priming and diluting solutions for CPB may consistently influence the fluid, chemical, humoral and homeostatic equilibria during CPB. Therefore, the following questions should be answered:

1. Can the priming solution affect the pathophysiology of CPB and so contribute to the outcome?
2. Is there an optimal priming solution?

According to Sackett, evidence based medicine is the conscientious, explicit and judicious use of the current best evidence from practice and research in making decisions about the care of individual patients [72]. Medical strategies shaped by non-evidence-based intuition and unsystematic clinical experience have to be abandoned.

There is a firm clinical demand for an appropriate substitution for blood and plasma during cardiac surgery with the special need to prime (i.e. fill up) the extracorporeal circuit. Natural colloids such as human albumin are extremely expensive, and there is little evidence to support the routine use of albumin. Alterna-

Table 8.1. Qualities of an ideal priming solution

No transmission of diseases (virus, bacterium, prion)
Sufficient and prolonged oncotic activity
Limited survival (transient but profound hemodilution)
No (or minimal) interference with: acid-base management; hemostasis; renal function; mediator release and complement (SIRS); metabolism
No anaphylaxis or anaphylactoid reactions
Reasonable cost

tives such as pure crystalloids and cheaper artificial colloids with different characteristics are available. The theoretical requirements for an ideal prime are summarized in Table 8.1.

Methods

A set of evaluated studies was produced from electronic databases related to this topic and by hand searching of selected journals and articles. From 1964 to 1997, there were about 225 references. Twenty-one randomized clinical studies were selected for more extensive review [1, 9, 14, 22, 29, 31, 33, 35, 36, 41, 43, 49, 54, 56, 57, 58, 62, 73, 75, 77, 80]. From this group, 11 studied albumin or plasma protein solution while nine evaluated starches, four compared a gelatin solution, and two studied dextran. Two studies were selected that compare exclusively crystalloids. The discussion is devoted to these papers and to some specific issues and additional points to illustrate the evidence.

Discussion

Colloid vs Crystalloid

Most studies comparing crystalloids with colloids found more positive fluid balances with crystalloids [33, 35, 36, 49, 54, 73]. However, clinical differences are not always considered important

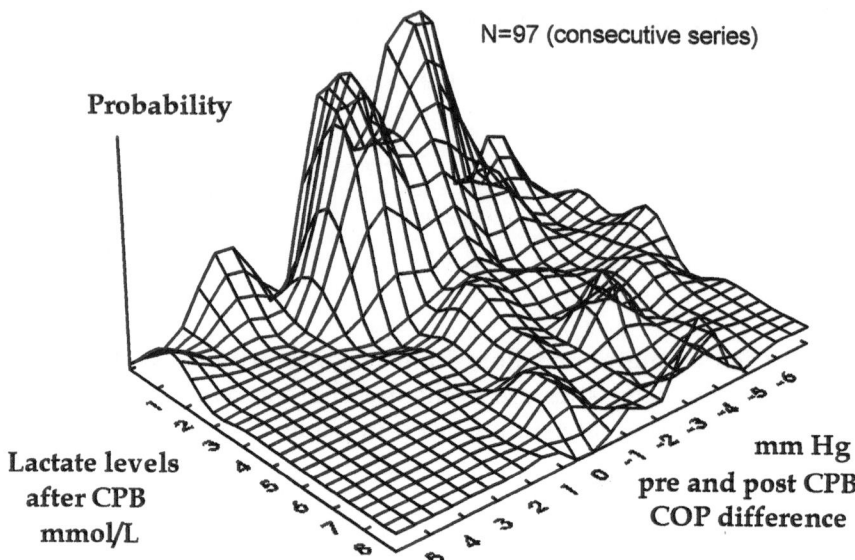

N=97 (consecutive series)

Probability

Lactate levels
after CPB
mmol/L

mm Hg
pre and post CPB
COP difference

Fig. 8.1. Three-dimensional surface of the relationship between post-bypass lactate levels and colloid oncotic pressure (COP) changes during cardiopulmonary bypass (CPB) using a non-protein colloidal prime (gelatin). The multi-modal chain of upward sloping in the back represents slightly elevated post-bypass lactate levels in most cases. There is an equal spread in both the positive and the negative directions starting from a zero difference in oncotic pressure before and after CPB. In firm contrast, the front shows smaller probability peaks associated with more elevated lactate levels, which are exclusively observed in the area corresponding with oncotic pressure differences less than zero (p=0.038; Student t-test). This is apparent from the left-to-right diffuse upward sloping in the front part of the graph

enough to advise the general use of colloids: crystalloids can also do the job in less risky routine patients [33, 36, 49, 54]. By contrast, adding a colloid is recommended for selected cases only in two studies [33, 54]. London concluded that both crystalloids and colloids are of equal value [49]. However, in a pro-con debate [48], the author proved to be a definite proponent and defender of colloids in the prime. Abboth found an important increase of intra-ocular pressure with crystalloid primes but not with a plasma protein solution [1]. Colloids have a favorable effect on fluid balances. If indicated, albumin seems to be the colloid of choice, but its use should be limited because of the expense [33, 54, 48].

Nevertheless, Jansen also found improved postoperative courses and a reduction in hospital stay using a succinylated gelatin colloid [35]. Moreover, the importance of maintaining a normal COP during CPB was underlined. The relevance of this is also illustrated in Fig. 8.1, showing the relationship between a decline of COP during bypass and high post-CPB lactate levels [30].

Moreover, excessive fluid gain and overload after cardiac surgery are not benign problems as they are accompanied by significant increases in postoperative morbidity and mortality [50]. Thus, adding a colloid to the prime seems to be mandatory [35, 73].

Protein vs Non-protein Colloid

As the prime contributor (70%–80%) to the plasma COP, albumin is important for fluid homeostasis of the systemic circulation. Albumin levels do not always correlate well with COP in critically ill patients [51]. Both intravascular and extravascular (reserve) pools of albumin represent, respectively, 40% and 60% of the total body content. Major surgical procedures are associated with significant changes in albumin distribution [51]. However, due to its slow half-life, restoration of albumin deficits cannot readily occur during the peri-operative period. Hypo-albuminemia is also accepted as a biological marker and risk indicator of metabolic stress in acutely ill patients [65]. Unfortunately, inductive reasoning from these aforementioned associations and observations has led to a simplistic response in patient care: increase serum albumin or protein levels to normal by use of exogenous human albumin [8]. Even its numerous transport and vehicle functions do not provide a rationale for its therapeutic use [51]. Maintenance of the COP can also be achieved by using cheap and harmless synthetic colloids. Only few data are available from comparative studies of colloid use during CPB [29, 49, 62, 73, 75]. Starch solutions are associated with increased bleeding risk [62, 73, 75]. Apart from that artificial colloids are considered equivalent to albumin or even better [29, 49, 73, 75]. Thus, not all synthetic colloids are of equal value [6, 60, 90] and significant differences in biological performance have been observed [64, 86–88].

Acid-Base Balance: Buffers

Currently, acid-base regulation without temperature correction (the „a-stat mode") is favored, according to Rahn [66]. Hence, in particular cerebral and myocardial cell function should be better preserved [82, 83]. In spite of many publications on acid-base management strategies, no definite information is available about the specific influence of different priming solutions and their contribution to the ease of maintaining the desired acid-base. Some investigators even report on their failure to obtain true a-stat or pH-stat conditions [4]. Himpe and collaborators showed that a succinyl-linked gelatin prime dissolved in a crystalloid vehicle containing lactate is more apt to obtain true a-stat conditions than urea-linked gelatin (polygeline) in saline or albumin in Hartmann [29]. Unfortunately, it has not been determined how rigorously pH and base-excess levels should be kept near the normal values to maintain the beneficial effects of the a-stat regulation. Furthermore, McKnight and co-workers suggest that lactate primes should not be employed in CPB because of their potential gluconeogenic effects and the potential dangers of hyperglycemia in cerebral ischemia [56]. On the other hand, adding sodium bicarbonate to prevent acidosis may precipitate calcium carbonate [37, 91]. Acetate, a bicarbonate precursor like lactate, significantly decreases systemic vascular resistance during CPB [84]. The efficacy and relevance of using buffers such as acetate, tham-acetate, and gluconate to realize true a-stat conditions in hypothermic CPB still have to be studied.

Glucose

Current evidence strongly supports the notion that hyperglycemia is likely to be detrimental to a brain challenged by ischemia, especially when there is reperfusion due to hypotension or circulatory arrest during normothermia [3, 32]. The avoidance of hyperglycemia during CPB seems prudent at present. In particular, the use of hypothermia during CPB results in higher blood glucose levels

[45]. Apart from reduced perioperative fluid requirements [58], the benefits of glucose are unknown and the probable risk to the central nervous system (CNS) is high. However, the contention that hyperglycemia exacerbates CNS deficits after cardiac operation has not been documented. Therefore, Metz concludes that, because embolism is the cause of most postoperative neurologic deficits, any increased risk due to hyperglycemia is small [59]. In contrast, McKnight firmly warns against using a glucose prime because of the danger of hyperglycemia [56]. Consequently, the advantages of glucose-containing CPB priming solutions are limited.

Coagulation and Platelet Function

Excessive bleeding during and after cardiac surgery with CPB is a real problem. Kutuinen advises not using starches in the CPB prime because of the increased risk for bleeding [43]. Furthermore, the effects of dextran [11, 61] and starch solutions [43, 62, 75, 87, 88] on coagulation have been extensively demonstrated requiring dose limits to be recommended. Cope recently recommended the avoidance of starches during cardiac surgery because of the impairment of hemostasis [16]. Boldt and co-workers have demonstrated that just crystalloid priming, the addition of hydroxyethyl starch or even high-dose albumin had significantly less beneficial effect on platelet function than gelatin or a combined solution of Ringer's, dextrose, and low-dose albumin [9].

Renal Function

In animal studies, Utley found that albumin causes decreased urine flow and diminished renal osmolar, sodium, and free-water clearances. Mannitol had no significant effect on urine flow, renal plasma flow, or renal clearances [89]. Most clinical studies failed to demonstrate any important difference in renal function or an inverse relationship with the COP during CPB in humans [47]. Dextrans and starches are also potentially deleterious [21, 81]. By contrast, gelatins seem to have no adverse effects on kidney function [40, 60].

The Systemic Inflammatory Response Syndrome

Activation of complement is a consistent phenomenon during CPB surgery and is associated with morbidity after CPB. Mellbye, comparing dextran and plasma as CPB primes, found the increase in complement activation products after CPB to be significantly higher in the plasma group than in the dextran group [57]. However, manipulation of the prime by using gelatins may reduce complement activation more than any other solution during CPB [25, 67]. Addition of a gelatin to the priming solution may be an inexpensive way of reducing morbidity [10].

Free Radical Scavengers

Some agents are thought to be able to scavenge oxygen-derived free radicals during ischemia and reperfusion. These include mannitol [63], dextrans [79], and perhaps also the other colloids. Stamler found that pentastarch produced fewer lung derangements than did a crystalloid prime, and no significant additional benefit was demonstrated with pentastarch conjugated to the free-radical scavenger deferoxamine [80]. No other comparative studies or clinical evidence on the efficacy of scavengers in CPB are available.

Coating of the Cardiopulmonary Bypass Circuit

Hemocompatible biomaterials are diverse with regard to both their origin and their physicochemical characteristics. None of them is ideal, and they ultimately produce local reactions (foreign body reactions, thrombosis) and systemic inflammatory reactions. Circuit-coating with heparin or other substances may offer some benefits. The addition of albumin to the prime was reported to increase biocompatibility by coating biomaterials [2, 9]. A similar beneficial blood-surface interaction has been demonstrated for gelatins [13].

Priming as a (Re-)Perfusate

Priming fluids also have a role as a perfusate when reperfusion occurs after clamping of aorta, hypotension, circulatory arrest or hypoperfusion during CPB. Christlieb, in a study on dogs, clearly demonstrated that adding a colloid to the prime is far more important for cardiac performance after release of the clamp than the choice of the cardioplegic solution [14]. Furthermore, Beards and Edwards and co-workers suggested that systemic organ reperfusion of critically ill patients in hypovolemic shock resulted in much better oxygen delivery to the tissues when gelatin was used as a resuscitation fluid instead of starch [7].

Rheology

Studies done on red blood cell (RBC) aggregation suggest that albumin and dextran 40 are superior to other colloids, with gelatin having a very weak score [5, 23]. RBC aggregation with rouleau formation is an important contributor to the increase of viscosity in low flow states in the presence of normal hematocrit levels. However, during hemodilution the relative importance of this phenomenon is far less [26], and, no comparative clinical studies are available that address this topic in the setting of CPB.

Addition of Ions: Potassium, Calcium, Magnesium

Supplementation of potassium during CPB is very common to maintain concentrations within the physiological range. Energy requirements of the heart are related to the ionized calcium concentration. Low plasma levels during CPB are considered advantageous for preventing the calcium-paradox phenomenon during reperfusion of the heart [19, 20]. When the heart takes over the circulating work, a normalization of the free calcium levels can be recommended [24] even though a temporary diastolic dysfunction may occur [17]. Routine addition of calcium supplements should be avoided [39, 42]. However, the importance of magnesium supplements in cardiac surgery cannot be overemphasized for its beneficial effect on the brain and on both heart rhythm and function [34, 38, 55].

Adverse Reactions

Significant anaphylactic or anaphylactoid reactions can occur. Except for dextran 60/70 and urea-linked gelatin, Ring and Messmer found no statistically significant differences between grade III and grade IV reactions [69]. Since then hapten prophylaxis of dextran reactions has been introduced, and the production process of urea-linked gelatin has been changed. More recently, Laxenaire and co-workers reported on the incidence of allergic reactions to colloids [44]. If only the life-threatening grades III and IV reactions are concerned no statistically significant differences were found. Furthermore, the calculated statistical power for the differences between starches and gelatins ranges only around 30%. Consequently, definitive conclusions cannot be drawn. Larger sample sizes are needed to demonstrate differences, in particular between the risks of grades III and IV reactions, if they exist [28].

End-Point Definition (Outcome)

Controversies about the priming with regard to outcome can be explained by the inability to define clearly comparable end-points [71]. Except for the extent of hemodilution in relation to neurological outcome [76, 78] no data are available about the composition of the priming solutions. Quantitative measuring of the extent to which a solution interferes with the pathophysiological mechanisms is difficult. Jansen showed a more than basic interest in outcome and developed a unique outcome score to estimate the inflammatory response which proved to be predictive for the hospital stay [35]. However, studies comparing true end-points like rates of myocardial infarction, neurological adverse effects, and mortality need more than 5000 subjects to demonstrate differences between 1% and 2% with a power of 80% [18].

Conclusions

This review identified a limited sample of the literature comparing CPB priming solutions. Although the assimilation is easy, it probably cannot be expected to provide sufficient evidence. Not all aspects of cardiac interventions with CPB are capable of being reduced to well-defined issues. Sometimes clinical artistry and individual experience are required to reach a good resolution. However, this exercise has taught us that there is objective evidence to support the argument that a colloid should be used in the CPB prime. An adequate and safe alternative to human albumin is succinylated gelatin, which is preferred. It is associated with a lower risk of bleeding and renal problems, and its cost is substantially less than that of albumin. In spite of its short half life, gelatin has the strongest affinity for water of all the colloids [52]. Therefore, it is the optimal solution for priming cardiopulmonary bypass machines to produce short-acting but very pronounced hemodilution with a minimal fluid gain. It is inexpensive and free of detrimental side effects. As long the manufacturer can guarantee the complete elimination of all protein fractions during its production, gelatin is safe and without risk of transmitting disease [53]. The addition of lactate may help to achieve a-stat conditions easier. However, lactate may increase glycemia, which has been associated with unfavorable outcomes after global brain ischemia. The exact levels of harmful glycemia during CPB have not yet been defined. More prospective, controlled clinical trials will be necessary to find out which are the best additives for the crystalloid vehicle and to establish all the effects of different colloids on organs and body systems. Since we are moving towards an era of normothermic CPB, the use of artificial oxygen carriers might be justified. These products can maintain sufficient oxygen transport to bridge the transient expansion of the circulating volume. And, finally, perhaps minimally invasive techniques may make CPB obsolete and terminate this discussion.

CHAPTER 9

Colloid-Induced Renal Complications 9

J.-F. BARON

Introduction

Normovolemic hemodilution with colloids is recommended in a wide range of ischemic conditions, such as acute stroke, peripheral vascular disease, and hearing loss, to improve microcirculatory perfusion and collateral flow. Since these patients usually have generalized atherosclerosis, often with some degree of preexisting latent renal disease, it is not surprising that the colloids, albumin, dextran, and HES are occasionally associated with the development of acute renal failure, particularly if dosage recommendations are not followed [1]. Several publications have recently focused on another category of patients at risk, brain-dead donors for kidney transplantation [2].

Acute Renal Failure Following Infusion of Colloids

This complication was initially described only with dextrans. In certain groups, particularly patients at high risk, such as those with acute stroke or stage III/IV arteritis, the reported incidence of acute renal failure associated with dextran therapy range from virtually 0% in the 500 patients on dextran 40 reported by Gottstein [3] to 4.3% in the 207 patients reported by Biesenbach [1]. The only evident, but possibly decisive, difference in these two reports concerns hydration: Gottstein's patients received an additional 250 ml 20% of mannitol plus at least 7000 ml crystalloids or oral water daily to maintain adequate urine output.

A review of 23 published case reports published by Matheson [4] suggests that most cases of colloid-induced acute renal failure share several risk factors: they were generally elderly patients; they had received colloids for nonsurgical reasons, claudication, stroke, or sudden hearing loss; they had preexisting or latent renal disease; they had been dehydrated with low urine output prior to colloid administration; and they had received high doses of 10% dextran 40 for several days.

Several hypotheses have been formulated to explain acute renal failure following dextran administration: direct toxicity, accumulation of low molecular weight fractions in the tubule, and more recently hyperoncotic renal failure.

Low molecular weight dextran is a mixture of dextrose polymers with an average molecular weight of 40,000 (range 10,000–80,000). In normal subjects the components with the lowest molecular weight are excreted by the kidney within 12–24 h while the largest components may be retained in plasma or interstitial compartments for weeks. The chemical toxicity of dextran is low although it may induce vacuolization of proximal tubular cells [5]. These osmotic nephrosis-like lesions have been reported with other colloids such as hydroxyethyl starches (HES) [6] and gelatins [7]. Initially these lesions were considered responsible for impairment in renal function; however, these have also been observed with drugs that do not induce acute renal failure as mannitol and glucose [7].

Mailloux et al. maintain that direct toxicity is unlikely since in laboratory animals dextran can induce acute renal failure within minutes after it is administered [8, 9]. In this setting, however, a prerequisite for the development of renal failure is severe constriction of the renal artery or severe hypovolemia as a consequence of noncompensated blood withdrawal. Mailloux et al. suggest that the combination of decreased glomerular pressure and maximal reabsorption of water induces the accumulation in the tubule of low molecular weight fraction of dextran with local hyperviscosity and precipitation.

Ten years later a case report by Moran et al. demonstrated the reversibility of acute renal failure by plasmapheresis [10]; this observation has been confirmed by several other publications [11–14]. This has led to the formulation of another explanation for colloid-induced acute renal failure, the hyperoncotic mechanism. The initial case report of Moran et al. demonstrated that a high plasma concentration of dextrans inducing a high plasma colloido-osmotic pressure counteracts the opposing hydraulic filtration pressure in the glomerulus. Indeed, the rate of glomerular filtration is governed by the imbalance between positive hydraulic forces that promote fluid movement into Bowman's space and negative oncotic forces that retard such movement [15, 16].

The glomerular filtration rate (GFR) may be expressed as GFR= K_f ($\Delta P - \Delta \Pi$) where K_f is the glomerular ultrafiltration coefficient, ΔP is the mean difference in hydraulic pressure, and $\Delta \Pi$ is the mean difference in oncotic pressure. Because glomerular filtrate is essentially free of protein, the value for $\Delta \Pi$ is determined primarily by oncotic pressure within the glomerular capillary. Acute renal failure induced by ischemia or cellular toxin is characterized by alterations in glomerular hemodynamics. Net transglomerular hydraulic pressure may be reduced either by a rise in proximal tubular pressure or by a fall in the hydraulic pressure in the glomerular capillary. Diminished glomerular permeability and tubuloglomerular feedback activation may also contribute to the reduction in the glomerular filtration rate [17]. Backleak of filtrate across a damaged tubular epithelium can further reduce renal excretory capacity [18]. The equation shows that glomerular filtration ceases if the oncotic forces equal or exceed the hydraulic forces. As protein-free glomerular filtrate is formed, the distal intracapillary oncotic pressure rises sufficiently to stop filtration [16]. Theoretically an accumulation in plasma of any unfilterable, osmotically active substance could likewise induce cessation of glomerular filtration.

Because pressure within the glomerular capillary and proximal tubule cannot actually be measured in humans, accurate determination of the minimal transcapillary hydraulic pressure required to form glomerular filtrate is difficult. The patient of Moran et al. [10] provided a unique opportunity to make such a calculation (Fig. 9.1). One can consider a hypothetical situation in which renal perfusion pressure is stable in the setting of anuria induced by elevated plasma oncotic pressure. If oncotic pressure is slowly reduced, urine flow returns when the net glomerular transcapillary hydraulic pressure just exceeds the oncotic pressure in the afferent

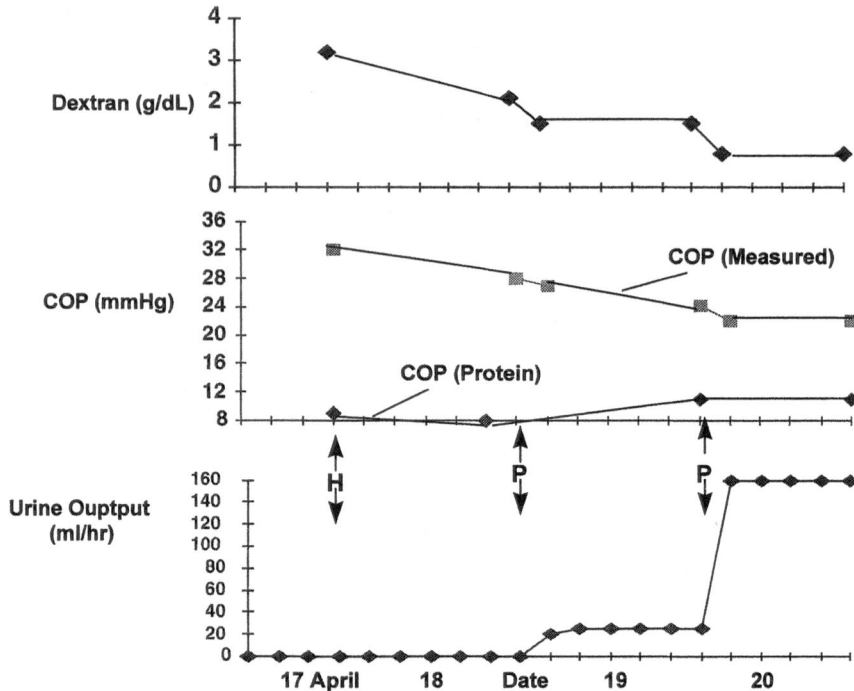

Fig. 9.1. Changes in dextran concentration, colloid osmotic pressure (*COP*) and urine output associated with hemodialysis and plasmapheresis (*P*). The last plasmapheresis demonstrates the mechanism of hyperoncotic acute renal failure. The patient had no urine output when the total oncotic pressure was 28.7 mmHg, and urine output returned when the oncotic pressure was 26.9 mmHg. Therefore a range of 27–29 mmHg probably encompassed the minimal value of the transmembrane difference in hydraulic pressure necessary to form glomerular filtrate. (From [10])

arteriole of patent nephrons. The patient had no urine output when the total oncotic pressure was 28.7 mmHg, and urine output returned when the oncotic pressure was 26.9 mmHg. Therefore a range of 27–29 mmHg probably encompassed the minimal value of the transmembrane difference in hydraulic pressure necessary to form glomerular filtrate.

This syndrome has been termed "hyperoncotic acute renal failure" [10]. The presence of anuria is not a diagnostic criterion. The patient's renal insufficiency developed over several days, initially during a period of nonoliguria. Presumably the nephrons became progressively nonfunctional. Such a sequence may occur commonly, with its cause mistakenly attributed to other factors. One can speculate that other subjects, such as those with hyperproteinemia, could also be at risk for hyperoncotic renal dysfunction.

This hypothesis has been reinforced by publication of additional cases following not only dextran but HES [19], gelatin [20], and concentrated albumin [21] administration. Most of these cases have also confirmed the beneficial effect of plasmapheresis [11, 12, 14]. Until recently hydroxyethyl starch was thought to be relatively free of these problems in conjunction with its use in hemodilution. In the past few years, however, the German Health Authority began receiving several reports which also implicated HES in this context [19]. It is now known that all hyperoncotic colloid solutions, 20% albumin [21], 10% HES 200 [19], and 10% dextran 40, can induce acute renal failure. Acute renal failure has also been documented with 6% hetastarch [22] and 3.5% gelatin [20] but not for 6% dextran 70, 3% dextran 60, or 5% albumin. It is likely that the risk of high plasma colloido-osmotic pressure is greater with colloids having either a high concentration (dextran 10%, HES 10%) or a high in vivo molecular weight responsible for plasma accumulation (hetastarch and elohes 6%).

In patients receiving colloids, particularly those with obstructive vascular disease, daily postoperative assessment of renal function is prudent. If renal function deteriorates and oligoanuria that is unresponsive to diuretic treatment occurs, direct measurement of colloid osmotic pressure is indicated. If the pressure is disproportionately elevated, the infusion of colloids should be stopped. If the decline in renal function is progressive, plasmapheresis may be the appropriate therapy.

Adverse Effects of Colloids on Transplanted Organs

In 1993 Legendre et al. reported osmotic nephrosis-like lesions in most of the transplanted kidneys subsequently biopsied at Necker Hospital in Paris [6]. In an historical study they found that 80% of the kidney transplanted at their center during 1992, when routine administration of HES was used with brain-dead donors, had osmotic nephrosis-like lesions in biopsies taken 6 weeks after transplantation. Only 14% of the kidneys transplanted in 1990, prior to the introduction of HES administration, revealed such lesions upon biopsy. Demographic data, the use of contrast media, and choice of preservation solution were similar in the two groups. The incidence of osmotic nephrosis-like lesions was not affected by cold ischemia time, presence and length of delayed graft function, or immunosuppressive regimen, especially the use of cyclosporine. Conversely, these lesions had no significant deleterious effect on the occurrence of delayed graft function and serum creatinine 3 and 6 months after transplantation. However, osmotic nephrosis-like lesions may be long-lasting since in three patients they were still present 3 months after transplantation on routine renal biopsy. In the patients without osmotic nephrosis-like lesions no kidney was lost, whereas 7 of 31 among those with such lesions were lost. Legendre et al. then recommended the avoidance of HES in potential organ donors.

Although accepting that the adverse effect on renal transplant survival is a new finding, the German Drug Committee decided that evidence is still insufficient to issue an official drug alert. They claimed that Legendre's publication, upon which the warning was based, is a retrospective case report analysis without statistical evaluation and therefore lacks scientific value.

A prospective randomized study was then carried out by Cittanova et al. [2] to determine the effects on renal function in kidney transplant recipient of administering HES or gelatin to brain-dead donors. Over 18 months 121 brain-dead donors were admitted in their hospital; those who had received iodinated contrast media were excluded. Multiple organ harvesting was possible in only 29, including 27 kidney donors, 15 in the HES group and 12 in the gelatin group, leading to, respectively, 27 and 20 kidney recipients in the HES group and gelatin group. In the HES group brain-dead patients needing colloids received HES up to the maximal dose of 33 ml/kg and then gelatin. In the gelatin group brain-dead donors received only gelatin for plasma volume expansion. There were no significant differences in age, cause or duration of brain-death, need for dopamine or other cardiovascular support, transfusion requirements, or preoperative serum creatinine between the two groups. One of 20 (5%) kidney recipients in the

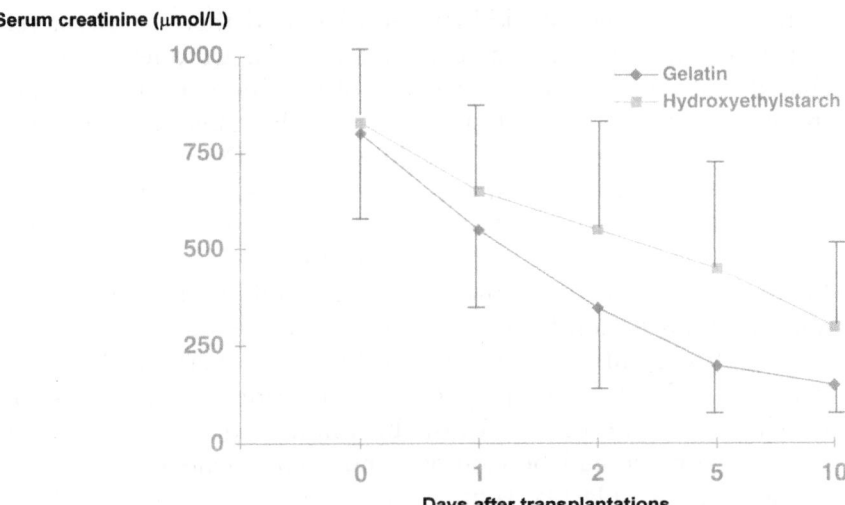

Fig. 9.2. Serum creatinine after kidney transplantation (mean±SD). (From [2])

gelatin group needed extrarenal hemodialysis or hemofiltration within the first week after transplantation, compared with 9 of 27 (33%) in the HES group ($p<0.03$). Serum creatinine for the first 10 days after transplantation was significantly lower in the gelatin group than in the HES group (Fig. 9.2). Nine real biopsy specimens were examined, six of which were in the gelatin group. All three specimens in the HES group had osmotic nephrosis-like lesions. This prospective randomized study seems to confirm the results of the earlier study of Legendre et al.

However, Coronel et al. have reported controversial data [23]. They analyzed 24 renal transplant biopsy specimens taken 15 min after kidney reperfusion, which they classified into groups according to the use of HES or not for the resuscitation of the brain-dead donors. Four of 16 (25%) patients who received HES had osmotic nephrosis-like lesions and 2 of 8 (25%) who did not received HES. In addition, they observed no functional effect of HES administration on postoperative kidney graft function. In this study the osmotic nephrosis-like lesions were less frequent (25%) than those reported by Legendre and Cittanova. In the study by Coronel there was no specific reason to attribute the lesions to HES. Indeed, none of these three studies identified HES in the vacuoles seen on kidney biopsies, and thus no direct relationship with HES has yet been established. Coronel et al. concluded that the hemodynamic status of the donor is still central to the occurrence of these lesions. It was also suggested that high colloido-osmotic pressure following colloid administration is an important mechanism which may contribute to explaining acute renal failure after kidney transplantation. Plasma colloido-osmotic pressure in the recipient may be of critical value when renal perfusion pressure is compromised after ischemic-reperfusion lesions, and this information is never available in these studies.

In addition, all these studies are limited to very small number patients, and a large scale-study is still needed to enable definite conclusions to be drawn. Until the findings of such a study are available, one should be cautious and recommend not using HES or dextrans as plasma volume expanders in brain-dead donors and in kidney-transplant recipients.

Conclusions

Colloid-induced acute renal failure generally occurs in the following groups of patients: the elderly; those receiving colloids for nonsurgical reasons, claudication, stroke, or sudden hearing loss; those with preexisting or latent renal disease; those dehydrated with low urine output prior to colloid administration; and those receiving high doses of colloids for several days. It has been demonstrated that a high plasma concentration of colloids inducing a high plasma colloido-osmotic pressure counteracts the opposing hydraulic filtration pressure in the glomerulus. This syndrome is termed hyperoncotic acute renal failure.

Hyperoncotic acute renal failure was initially observed only with dextrans, but it is now known that all hyperoncotic colloid solutions, 20% albumin, 10% HES 200, and 10% dextran 40, can induce acute renal failure. Acute renal failure has also been documented for 6% hetastarch and gelatin but not for 6% dextran 70, 3% dextran 60, or 5% albumin. It is likely that the risk of high plasma colloido-osmotic pressure is higher with colloids having either a high concentration (dextran 10%, HES 200 10%, albumin

20%) or a high in vivo molecular weight responsible for plasma accumulation (hetastarch or elohes 6%).

In patients receiving colloids, particularly those with obstructive vascular disease, daily postoperative assessment of renal function is prudent. If renal function deteriorates, and oligoanuria unresponsive to diuretic treatment occurs, direct measurement of colloid osmotic pressure is indicated. If the pressure is disproportionately elevated, the infusion of colloids should be stopped. If the decline in renal function is progressive, plasmapheresis may be the appropriate therapy.

References

1. Biesenbach G, Kaiser W, Zazgornik J (1997) Incidence of acute oligoanuric renal failure in dextran 40 treated patients with acute ischemic stroke stage III or IV. Ren Fail 19 (1):69–75
2. Cittanova ML, Leblanc I, Legendre C, Mouquet C, Riou B, Coriat P (1996) Effect of hydroxyethylstarch in brain-dead kidney donors on renal function in kidney-transplant recipients. Lancet 348:1620–1622
3. Gottstein U (1974) Treatment of inadequate cerebral circulation. A critical review. Internist (Berl) 15 (12):575–587
4. Matheson NA, Diomi P (1970) Renal failure after the administration of dextran 40. Surg Gynecol Obstet 131 (4):661–668
5. Diomi P, Ericsson JL, Matheson NA (1970) Effects of dextran 40 on urine flow and composition during renal hypoperfusion in dogs with osmotic nephrosis. Ann Surg 172 (5):813–824
6. Legendre C, Thervet E, Page B, Percheron A, Noel LH, Kreis H (1993) Hydroxyethylstarch and osmotic-nephrosis-like lesions in kidney transplantation. Lancet 342:248–49
7. Kief H (1969) Morphological findings following single or multiple administration of gelatin plasma substitutes. Bibl Haematol 33:367–379
8. Mailloux L, Swartz CD, Capizzi R, Kim KE, Onesti G, Ramirez O, Brest AN (1967) Acute renal failure after administration of low-molecular weight dextran. N Engl J Med 277 (21):1113–1118
9. Chinitz JL, Kim KE, Onesti G, Swartz C (1971) Pathophysiology and prevention of dextran-40-induced anuria. J Lab Clin Med 77 (1):76–87
10. Moran M, Kapsner C (1987) Acute renal failure associated with elevated plasma oncotic pressure. N Engl J Med 317 (3):150–153
11. Ferraboli R, Malheiro PS, Abdulkader RC, Yu L, Sabbaga E, Burdmann EA (1997) Anuric acute renal failure caused by dextran 40 administration. Ren Fail 19 (2):303–306

12. Kurnik BR, Singer F, Groh WC (1991) Case report: dextran-induced acute anuric renal failure. Am J Med Sci 302 (1):28–30
13. Zwaveling JH, Meulenbelt J, van Xanten NH, Hene RJ (1989) Renal failure associated with the use of dextran-40. Neth J Med 35 (5–6):321–326
14. Van Den Berg CJ, Pineda AA (1980) Plasma exchange in the treatment of acute renal failure due to low molecular-weight dextran. Mayo Clin Proc 55 (6):387–389
15. Myers BD (1983) Pathogenesis of acute renal failure in man. Kidney 16:37–41
16. Deen WM, Robertson CR, Brenner BM (1972) A model of glomerular ultrafiltration in the rat. Am J Physiol 223 (5):1178–1183
17. Stein JH (1977) The glomerulus in acute renal failure. J Lab Clin Med 90 (2):227–230
18. Blantz RC, Pelayo JC (1984) A functional role for the tubuloglomerular feedback mechanism. Kidney Int 25 (5):739–746
19. Waldhausen P, Kiesewetter H, Leipnitz G, Scielny J, Jung F, Bambauer R, von Blohn G (1991) Hydroxyethyl starch-induced transient renal failure in preexisting glomerular damage. Acta Med Austriaca 1:52–55
20. Hussain SF, Drew PJ (1989) Acute renal failure after infusion of gelatins. BMJ 299:1137–1138
21. Rozich JD, Paul RV (1989) Acute renal failure precipitated by elevated colloid osmotic pressure. Am J Med 87 (3):359–360
22. Haskell LP, Tannenberg AM (1988) Elevated urinary specific gravity in acute oliguric renal failure due to hetastarch administration. NY State J Med 88 (7):387–388
23. Coronel B, Mercatello A, Martin X, Lefrancois N (1997) Hydroxyethylstarch and renal function in kidney transplant recipients. Lancet 349:884

CHAPTER 10

New Therapeutic Concepts Using Artificial   10
Oxygen Carriers

D. R. Spahn

Introduction

Artificial oxygen (O_2) carriers aim at improving O_2 transport and O_2 unloading to the tissue. Artificial O_2 carriers thus may be used as an alternative to allogeneic blood transfusions or to improve tissue oxygenation and the function of organs with marginal O_2 supply. The aim of the present article is to describe the artificial O_2 carriers that have currently been evaluated, to summarize their efficiency and to discuss potential side effects.

The artificial O_2 carriers that have been evaluated to date can be grouped into modified hemoglobin solutions and fluorocarbon emulsions (Table 10.1). The native human hemoglobin molecule needs to be modified in order to decrease O_2 affinity and to prevent rapid dissociation of the native $a2–\beta2$ tetramer into $a–\beta$ dimers. This has been reviewed in detail previously [1].

The O_2-transport characteristics of modified hemoglobin solutions and fluorocarbon emulsions are fundamentally different

Table 10.1. Artificial O_2 carriers. The modified hemoglobin solutions are grouped by the source of the hemoglobin

Modified hemoglobin solutions
  Outdated human blood
  Bovine hemoglobin
  Human recombinant hemoglobin
    E. coli [36]
    Transgenic tabacco [37]
Fluorocarbon emulsions
  Perflubron

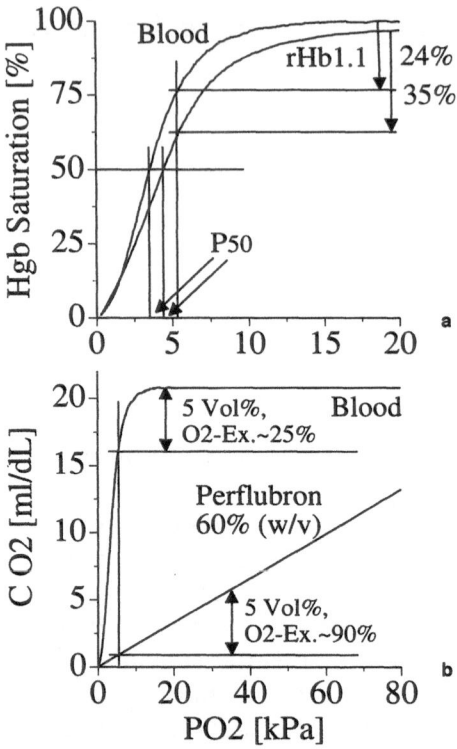

Fig. 10.1. a O_2 dissociation curve of native human blood (*Blood*) and human recombinant hemoglobin version 1.1 (*rHb1.1*) (modified according to Looker et al. [36]). P50 = partial O_2 pressure required for a 50% O_2 saturation. Note the higher P50 (4.4 kPa) resulting in a greater O_2 unloading capacity (35%) for rHb1.1 compared with native blood (P50=3.5 kPa and O_2 unloading capacity of 24%), when assuming a mixed venous PO_2 of 5.3 kPa. **b** O_2-carrying capacity of native human blood (Blood) and Perflubron (modified according to Keipert et al. [28]). Note that 5 vol% of O_2 can be unloaded by blood as well as by Perflubron. With Perflubron, however, higher arterial PO_2 values are required. Note also that Perflubron-transported O_2 is more completely unloaded than blood-transported O_2 resulting in approximate O_2 extraction (O_2-ex.) ratios of 90% and 25%. CO_2 denotes O_2 content and PO_2 denotes O_2 partial pressure

(Fig. 10.1). The modified hemoglobin solutions exhibit a sigmoidal O_2 dissociation curve similar to that of blood. In contrast, the fluorocarbon emulsions are characterized by a linear relationship between O_2 partial pressure and O_2 content. Modified hemoglobin solutions thus provide O_2 transport and unloading capacities similar to those of blood. This means that even at a relatively low arterial O_2 partial pressure substantial amounts of O_2 are being transported. In contrast, relatively high arterial O_2 partial pressures are necessary to maximize the O_2-transport capacity of fluorocarbon emulsions. Despite these fundamental differences, the efficiency of both groups of artificial O_2 carriers has been proven in a variety of experimental conditions (see below).

Hemoglobin Solutions

The efficiency of hemoglobin solutions in transporting and unloading O_2 has been shown in a variety of shock models and at extreme hemodilution (referenced in [1]; Table 10.2). In a whole animal sheep model, Vlahakes et al. [2] showed in awake sheep that extreme hemodilution to a hematocrit of 2.4±0.5% was only tolerated when a polymerized bovine hemoglobin solution was used, but not in animals treated with hydroxyethyl starch devoid of O_2-carrying capacity. All animals surviving acute hemodilution also survived the following 25 days without evidence of renal or hepatic dysfunction [2]. Similar results were achieved recently when the blood of anesthetized dogs was hemodiluted to a hematocrit of 2.0±1.8% using a polymerized bovine hemoglobin solution [3]. Even at this extremely low hematocrit, the dogs were hemodynamically stable, there was no evidence of (lactic) acidosis and there were no histologic signs of ultrastructural destruction in liver and kidney.

Siegel at al. [4] found in dogs that infusion of human recombinant hemoglobin (rHb1.1) resulted in a more rapid reversal of O_2 deficit after progressive hemorrhage, a more uniform reperfusion and a more complete wash-out of acids accumulated during build-up of the O_2 debt during hemorrhage compared with treatment with a mixture of autologous blood and colloid.

In a rat model of hemorrhage and surgical trauma, Xu et al. [5] furthermore demonstrated that treatment with a-a-Diaspirin cross-linked hemoglobin improved wound healing, enhanced hepatic cell proliferation and, most importantly, decreased splanch-

Table 10.2. Hemoglobin solutions: advantages and disadvantages

Advantages	Disadvantages
Carries and unloads O_2 Sigmoidal O_2 dissociation curve 100% FiO_2 is not mandatory for maximal potency Easy to measure	Side effects: Vasoconstriction Interference with colorimetric laboratory methods

nic bacterial translocation when compared with transfusion of fresh autologous blood. It is of particular interest that treatment with a-a-Diaspirin cross-linked hemoglobin induced a more favorable response to trauma and hemorrhage than transfusion of fresh autologous blood, considering the fact that the efficacy of blood transfusions in improving O_2 consumption and aerobic metabolism is not exactly defined [6]. In fact, only fresh blood (3 days old) but not 28-day-old blood was recently shown to partially correct the decrease in O_2 consumption induced by extreme hemodilution [7]. It is therefore particularly noteworthy that a-a-Diaspirin was even more effective than a transfusion of fresh autologous blood that was not stored at all [5].

Bovine polymerized hemoglobin was also more efficient in restoring muscle PO_2 after extreme hemodilution to a hematocrit of 10% in dogs than fresh (day of experiment) or old (21 days) autologous blood [8]. Likewise, muscle PO_2 was better restored with bovine polymerized hemoglobin than hydroxyethyl starch in a dog model of hemodilution (hematocrit of 23%–27%) and 95% arterial stenosis [9].

Hemoglobin solutions have also been used in resuscitation from hemorrhagic shock [10]. In awake sheep bled to a base deficit of –5 to –10 mEq/L, infusion of a-a-Diaspirin cross-linked hemoglobin restored base deficit at a similar rate as the infusion of autologous blood. Thereby, blood and a-a-Diaspirin cross-linked hemoglobin both were significantly more efficient than hydroxyethyl starch, a colloid without O_2-carrying capacity.

Thus, modified hemoglobin solutions are indeed very promising in improving O_2 transport and tissue oxygenation to a physiologically relevant degree. Without the need for cross matching, these solutions thus hold great promise as an alternative to allo-geneic blood transfusions and as O_2 treatments which may also be of great value in the prehospital resuscitation of trauma victims or in specific situations in intensive care medicine.

Since the breakdown of the native $a2$-$\beta2$ hemoglobin tetramer into a-β dimers is largely prevented by genetic modification or chemical modification, nephrotoxicity is no longer a potential side effect of these solutions [11]. Simultaneously, intravascular half-life was also prolonged. Interestingly, intravascular half life in-creases with increasing dose [12] (for a-a-Diaspirin cross-linked hemoglobin) and increases with achieved plasma hemoglobin concentration [11] (human recombinant hemoglobin, rHbl.1). Although there are no definitive data available on the intravascu-lar half-life of the various modified hemoglobin solutions in hu-mans, a dose-related increase in intravascular half-life could be very advantageous for the clinical use of these substances.

Vasoconstriction resulting in an increase in systemic and pul-monary artery pressures has been observed with all modified he-moglobin solutions evaluated so far. The mechanisms involved in-clude nitric oxide (NO) scavenging [1, 13–15], endothelin release [16] and a sensitization of peripheral a adrenergic receptors [17]. NO scavenging has been the subject of a variety of studies [1, 13, 15]. NO produced by the endothelial cells is intended to react with the Fe^{2+} in the guanylate cyclase located in the smooth mus-cle cells of the vessel wall to modulate the vascular tone towards vasodilatation. It has been speculated that, in particular, unpoly-merized hemoglobin molecules may penetrate into the interstitial space of the subendothelial layers of vessel walls [18]. Extravascu-lar hemoglobin at this location would be perfectly positioned to scavenge NO and thus to shift vasomotor tone towards vasocon-striction. Although, to my knowledge, there are no studies directly proving the presence of exogenous hemoglobin molecules within the interstitial space of blood vessels, there are studies document-ing the extravasation of hemoglobin molecules [19, 20].

Involvement of NO-scavenging in the vasopressor effect of many hemoglobin solutions is, furthermore, suggested by the particular efficiency of NO donors such as nitroglycerin and L-arginine in de-creasing hemoglobin-induced hypertension [21]. An increase in mean arterial pressure due to hemoglobin infusion could also be prevented with endothelin receptor antagonists [16]. Thus there are ways to prevent or treat hemoglobin-mediated vasoconstriction.

Hemoglobin-induced vasoconstriction may be regarded as an untoward side effect. This view may be correct when relatively small volumes of hemoglobin solutions are being given to patients with a reduced cardiac contractility and a normal or elevated mean arterial pressure. In such patients, a hemoglobin infusion may induce increases in systemic and pulmonary vascular resistances high enough to cause a reduction in cardiac output [14]. In contrast, in a previously healthy trauma victim suffering from severe hypovolemia due to massive hemorrhage, the combined effects of volume replacement, added O_2-transport capacity and a certain vasoconstriction due to the infusion of a modified hemoglobin solution may be very beneficial indeed. Very important in this regard is also the recent observation that the vasoconstriction due to a-a-Diaspirin cross-linked hemoglobin is not distributed evenly throughout the body. Dietz et al. [15] found that vasoconstriction was most pronounced in the femoral artery supplying mainly skeletal muscles but no vasoconstriction was observed in the mesenteric vasculature and a distinct vasodilatory effect was observed in the coronaries. Furthermore, hemoglobin-mediated vasoconstriction may be used therapeutically in patients with septic shock to decrease the vasopressor support with norepinephrine [22].

Other aspects of hemoglobin solutions are worth mentioning. Since hemoglobin solutions are colored solutions, the potential exists for some colorimetric laboratory measurement methods to be disturbed [23]. There is also one report in dogs, in which infusion of human recombinant hemoglobin induced an increase in liver enzymes as well as amylase [4]. However, in other studies in which even larger quantities of bovine hemoglobin have been given, no hepatic dysfunction was observed during 25 days after near-complete exchange transfusion [2].

Fluorocarbon Emulsions

Fluorocarbons are carbon-fluorine compounds characterized by a high gas-dissolving capacity (O_2, CO_2 and other gases), low viscosity, and chemical and biologic inertness [1, 24] (Table 10.3). Fluorocarbons are virtually not miscible with water. The first generation fluorocarbons, such as Fluosol (Green Cross, Japan), used a poloxamer type Pluronic F-68 as an emulsifier, which, however, has the potential to cause anaphylaxis [24]. The second-generation fluorocarbons use egg-yolk phospholipide as emulsifier, which is well tolerated except in patients with an egg allergy [1, 24].

Manufacturing an emulsion with very specific characteristics is a great technological challenge because only droplets of a very specific size (around 0.2 μm in diameter) are well tolerated. The spectrum of side effects also critically depends on the size distribution of the droplets: the narrower the distribution around the target size, the lesser, in general, are the side effects. With the development of a stable 60% (58% perfluorooctyl bromide and 2% perfluorodecyl bromide) emulsion there is now a relatively highly concentrated emulsion which is clinically well tolerated [24, 25].

After intravenous administration, the droplets of the emulsion are taken up by the reticulo-endothelial system (RES). This uptake into the RES determines intravascular half-life [1, 24]. At the present time no exact data are yet available on the intravascular half life in humans. After the initial uptake of the fluorocarbon emulsion into the RES, the droplets are slowly broken down and the fluorocarbon molecules are taken up into the blood again (bound to blood lipids) and transported to the lungs, where the unaltered fluorocarbon molecules are finally excreted via exhalation. At the present time, metabolism of fluorocarbon molecules is unknown in humans [1, 24].

The ability of fluorocarbon emulsions to transport and efficiently unload O_2 is undisputed. Young et al. [26] showed in pa-

Table 10.3. Fluorocarbon emulsions: advantages and disadvantages

Advantages	Disadvantages
Carries and unloads O_2	100% FiO_2 is mandatory for maximal potency
Few and mild side effects	Additional colloid often necessary with potential side effects
No known organ toxicity	

tients undergoing coronary angioplasty that distal coronary perfusion with oxygenated Fluosol largely blunted myocardial lactate release during balloon inflation and prevented major regional wall motion abnormalities, resulting in a far better-preserved left ventricular ejection fraction. The ischemia-preventing effect of distal coronary perfusion with Fluosol was confirmed by Kent et al. [27], again demonstrating by echocardiography that wall motion was far better preserved during balloon inflation in transluminal coronary angioplasty and that patients experienced significantly less angina.

Perflubron was assessed in a variety of hemodilution studies. Keipert et al. [28] applied Perflubron in dogs after acute normovolemic hemodilution at a hematocrit of 10%. During hemodilution the expected increase in cardiac output was observed [1, 28]. With the administration of Perflubron, cardiac output tended to increase further and a massive rise in mixed venous O_2 partial pressure and mixed venous saturation was observed. The percentage of metabolized O_2 originating from endogenous hemoglobin decreased dramatically with the administration of Perflubron, indicating that the O_2 transported by Perflubron is preferentially metabolized, most likely due to the excellent O_2-unloading characteristics of this fluorocarbon emulsion [28].

Furthermore, Holman et al. [29] tested Perflubron in the severely hemodiluted blood of dogs undergoing cardiopulmonary bypass. Without the use of catecholamines, dogs treated with increasing doses of Perflubron survived cardiopulmonary bypass progressively better than control animals. In addition, brain tissue oxygenation may be improved by a combined treatment with Perflubon infusion and 100% oxygen ventilation, notably more than with 100% oxygen ventilation alone [30].

Perflubron may also be beneficial as an adjunct to resuscitation. In a porcine model of near-fatal hemorrhage, Perflubron treatment in addition to standard resuscitation decreased mortality from 43% to 13% [31]. Although this difference did not reach statistical significance due to a low number of observations ($n = 15$ total) it was felt by the authors that the added and readily available O_2 provided by Perflubron was beneficial. Also in a dog model of ventricular fibrillation the additional direct infusion of oxygenated Perflubron into the aortic arch improved the chances of spontaneous return of circulation and this was achieved earlier than with standard resuscitation [32].

Perflubron has also been used in humans [25]. Acute normovolemic hemodilution to a hemoglobin concentration of approximately 9 g/dl was performed preoperatively. During surgery, Perflubron (0.9 g/kg) was administered when a blood transfusion was deemed necessary by the anesthetist which occurred at a hemoglobin concentration of approximately 8 g/dl. Mixed venous oxygen tension and mixed venous oxygen saturation both increased significantly after Perflubron administration, and cardiac output was stable. Although only relatively little O_2 was transported by Perflubron (approximately 1%), 5% of the metabolized O_2 originated from Perflubron-transported O_2, again indicating that Perflubron-transported O_2 is preferentially metabolized [25, 28].

Fluorocarbon emulsions also have side effects. Volunteers experienced mild influenza-like symptoms with myalgia and light fever and an approximately 15% decrease in platelet count 3 days post-dosing, returning to normal by day 7 [24, 33]. Traditional coagulation tests including bleeding time, however, were unaffected by Perflubron [33]. With a modification of the fluorocarbon emulsion, these side effects were blunted and thus no longer represent a relevant clinical problem.

Comparison Between Hemoglobin Solutions and Fluorocarbon Emulsions

The direct comparison between hemoglobin solutions and fluorocarbon emulsions is difficult. To a large extent this is related to the fact that there are no comparative studies, either between different hemoglobin solutions or between hemoglobin solutions and fluorocarbon emulsions. Despite the lack of such direct comparisons, there are several aspects in which these substances indeed can be compared. In this comparison, qualitatively similar properties of the different hemoglobin solutions are assumed, although this assumption may not be correct.

Hemoglobin solutions are also isooncotic or even hyperoncotic colloidal volume expanders. Infusion of these solutions thus not only provides additional O_2-carrying and unloading capacity; these solutions will also correct hypovolemia. In contrast, the volume of fluorocarbon emulsions infused is relatively small with the doses currently used. Therefore, additional volume expanders have to be infused to correct hypervolemia. The more liberal use of additional volume expanders may render their side effects more clinically relevant. Amongst these side effects, the effect on blood coagulation may be particularly important. Egli et al. [34] have recently demonstrated that blood coagulation may indeed become compromised during advanced hemodilution and that there are relevant differences between gelatin, albumin and hydroxyethyl starch volume expanders.

Another clinical issue is the monitoring of the effectiveness of artificial O_2 carriers. This may seem to be particularly difficult for the fluorocarbon emulsions because there is no means of bedside measurement of the fluorocarbon concentration of fluorocrit available. In contrast, with hemoglobin solutions such a problem seems not to exist because regular laboratory measurement techniques do measure total hemoglobin, i.e., the sum of endogenous hemoglobin (within red blood cells) and exogenous hemoglobin (in the plasma) correctly. However, since we should not go by hemoglobin concentration alone in our decision regarding blood transfusions [35], the above difference may not be as relevant. However, the daily practice in many institutions is still to transfuse blood primarily based on institutional guidelines in which the hemoglobin concentration may be a crucial parameter. Also, the course used for the production of these solutions may matter for certain groups of physicians and patients, such as Jehovah's witnesses.

Knowledge about both categories of artificial O_2 carriers is not sufficient to favor one solution over another at the present time. Hemoglobin solutions as well as fluorocarbon emulsions have both proven in many situations to efficiently transport and unload O_2. Furthermore, it is expected that modified formulations will be developed which even better serve this purpose in the future. Artificial O_2 carriers are thus very promising substances which will enter clinical medicine within the next 5 years, most likely before the year 2000.

References

1. Spahn DR, Leone BJ, Reves JG, Pasch T (1994) Cardiovascular and coronary physiology of acute isovolemic hemodilution: a review of nonoxygen-carrying and oxygen-carrying solutions. Anesth Analg 78:1000–1021
2. Vlahakes GJ, Lee R, Jacobs EE, LaRaia PJ, Austen WG (1990) Hemodynamic effects and oxygen transport properties of a new blood substitute in a model of massive blood replacement. J Thorac Cardiovasc Surg 100:379–388
3. Standl T, Lipfert B, Reeker W, Schulte am Esch J, Lorke DE (1996) Akute Auswirkungen eines kompletten Blutaustauschs mit ultragereinigter Hämoglobinlösung oder Hydroxyäthylstärke auf Leber und Niere im Tiermodell. Anasthesiol Intensivmed Notfallmed Schmerzther 31:354–361
4. Siegel JH, Fabian M, Smith JA, Costantino D (1997) Use of recombinant hemoglobin solution in reversing lethal hemorrhagic hypovolemic oxygen debt shock. J Trauma 42:199–212
5. Xu L, Sun L, Rollwagen FM, Li Y, Pacheco ND, Pikoulis E, Leppaniemi A, Soltero R, Burris D, Malcolm D, Nielsen TB (1997) Cellular responses to surgical trauma, hemorrhage, and resuscitation with diaspirin cross-linked hemoglobin in rats. J Trauma 42:32–41
6. Hebert PC, Hu LQ, Biro GP (1997) Review of physiologic mechanisms in response to anemia. Can Med Assoc J 156:27-40
7. Fitzgerald RD, Martin CM, Dietz GE, Doig GS, Potter RF, Sibbald WJ (1997) Transfusing red blood cells stored in citrate phosphate dextrose adenine-1 for 28 days fails to improve tissue oxygenation in rats. Crit Care Med 25:726–732
8. Standl T, Horn P, Wilhelm S, Greim C, Freitag M, Freitag U, Sputtek A, Jacobs E, Schulte am Esch J (1996) Bovine haemoglobin is more potent than autologous red blood cells in restoring muscular tissue oxygenation after profound isovolaemic haemodilution in dogs. Can J Anaesth 43:714–723
9. Horn EP, Standl T, Wilhelm S, Jacobs EE, Freitag U, Freitag M, Esch JSA (1997) Bovine hemoglobin increases skeletal muscle oxygenation during 95 percent artificial arterial stenosis. Surgery 121:411–418
10. DeAngeles DA, Scott AM, McGrath AM, Korent VA, Rodenkirch LA, Conhaim RL, Harms BA (1997) Resuscitation from hemorrhagic shock with diaspirin cross-linked hemoglobin, blood, or hetastarch. J Trauma 42:406–412;
11. Viele MK, Weiskopf RB, Fisher D (1997) Recombinant human hemoglobin does not affect renal function in humans: analysis of safety and pharmacokinetics. Anesthesiology 86:848–858
12. Przybelski RJ, Daily EK, Kisicki JC, Mattia Goldberg C, Bounds MJ, Colburn WA (1996) Phase I study of the safety and pharmacologic effects of diaspirin cross-linked hemoglobin solution. Crit Care Med 24:1993–2000

13. Jia L, Bonaventura J, Stamler JS (1996) S-nitrosohaemoglobin: a dynamic activity of blood involved in vascular control. Nature 380:221–226
14. Kasper SM, Walter M, Grüne F, Bischoff A, Erasmi H, Buzello W (1996) Effects of a hemoglobin-based oxygen carrier (HBOC-201) on hemodynamics and oxygen transport in patients undergoing preoperative hemodilution for elective abdominal aortic surgery. Anesth Analg 83:921–927
15. Dietz NM, Martin CM, Beltrandelrio AG, Joyner MJ (1997) The effects of cross linked hemoglobin on regional vascular conductance in dogs. Anesth Analg 85:265–273
16. Gulati A, Sharma AC, Singh G (1996) Role of endothelin in the cardiovascular effects of diaspirin crosslinked and stroma reduced hemoglobin. Crit Care Med 24:137–147
17. Gulati A, Rebello S (1994) Role of adrenergic mechanisms in the pressor effect of diaspirin cross-linked hemoglobin J Lab Clin Med 124:125–133
18. Gould SA, Moss GS (1996) Clinical development of human polymerized hemoglobin as a blood substitute. World J Surg 20:1200–1207
19. Keipert PE, Gomez CL, Gonzales A, MacDonald VW, Hess JR, Winslow RM (1994) Diaspirin cross-linked hemoglobin: tissue distribution and long-term excretion after exchange transfusion. J Lab Clin Med 123:701–711
20. Bleeker WK, van der Plas J, Feitsma RI, Agterberg J, Rigter G, de Vries van Rossen A, Pauwels EK, Bakker JC (1989) In vivo distribution and elimination of hemoglobin modified by intramolecular cross-linking with 2-nor-2-formylpyridoxal 5'-phosphate. J Lab Clin Med 113:151–161
21. Schultz SC, Grady B, Cole F, Hamilton I, Burhop K, Malcolm DS (1993) A role for endothelin and nitric oxide in the pressor response to diaspirin cross-linked hemoglobin. J Lab Clin Med 122:301–308
22. Reah G, Bodenham AR, Mallick A, Daily EK, Przybelski RJ (1997) Initial evaluation of diaspirin cross-linked hemoglobin (DCLHb) as a vasopressor in critically ill patients. Crit Care Med 25:1480–1488
23. Ma Z, Monk TG, Goodnough LT, McClellan A, Gawryl M, Clark T, Moreira P, Keipert PE, Scott MG (1997) Effect of hemoglobin- and Perflubron-based oxygen carriers on common clinical laboratory tests. Clin Chem 43:1732–1737
24. Riess JG (1992) Overview of progress in the fluorocarbon approach to in vivo oxygen delivery. Biomater Artif Cells Immobil Biotechnol 20:183–202
25. Wahr JA, Trouwborst A, Spence RK, Henny CP, Cernaianu AC, Graziano GP, Tremper KK, Flaim KE, Keipert PE, Faithfull NS, Clymer JJ (1996) A pilot study of the effects of a perflubron emulsion, AF 0104, on mixed venous oxygen tension in anesthetized surgical patients. Anesth Analg 82:103–107
26. Young LH, Jaffe CC, Revkin JH, McNulty PH, Cleman M (1990) Metabolic and functional effects of perfluorocarbon distal perfusion during coronary angioplasty. Am J Cardiol 65:986–990
27. Kent KM, Cleman MW, Cowley MJ, Forman MB, Jaffe CC, Kaplan M, King SD, Krucoff MW, Lassar T, McAuley B, et al (1990) Reduction of

myocardial ischemia during percutaneous transluminal coronary angioplasty with oxygenated Fluosol. Am J Cardiol 66:279–284

28. Keipert PE, Faithfull NS, Bradley JD, Hazard DY, Hogan J, Levisetti MS, Peters RM (1994) Oxygen delivery augmentation by low-dose perfluorochemical emulsion during profound normovolemic hemodilution. Adv Exp Med Biol 345:197–204

29. Holman WL, Spruell RD, Ferguson ER, Clymer JJ, Vicente WV, Murrah CP, Pacifico AD (1995) Tissue oxygenation with graded dissolved oxygen delivery during cardiopulmonary bypass. J Thorac Cardiovasc Surg 110:774–785

30. van Rossem K, Vermarien H, Faithfull NS, Wouters L, Decuyper K (1997) Effects of perflubron emulsion and 100% oxygen breathing on local tissue PO_2 in brain cortex of unanaesthetized rabbits. Adv Exp Med Biol 411:403–409

31. Stern SA, Dronen SC, McGoron AJ, Wang X, Chaffins K, Millard R, Keipert PE, Faithfull NS (1995) Effect of supplemental perfluorocarbon administration on hypotensive resuscitation of severe uncontrolled hemorrhage. Am J Emerg Med 13:269–275

32. Manning JE, Batson DN, Payne FB, Adam N, Murphy CA, Perretta SG, Norfleet EA (1997) Selective aortic arch perfusion during cardiac arrest: enhanced resuscitation using oxygenated perflubron emulsion, with and without aortic arch epinephrine. Ann Emerg Med 29:580–587

33. Keipert PE, Faithfull NS, Roth DJ, Bradley JD, Batra S, Jochelson P, Flaim KE (1996) Supporting tissue oxygenation during acute surgical bleeding using a perfluorochemical-based oxygen carrier. Adv Exp Med Biol 388:603–9

34. Egli GA, Zollinger A, Seifert B, Popovic D, Pasch T, Spahn DR (1997) Effect of progressive haemodilution with hydroxyethyl starch, gelatin and albumin on blood coagulation. An in vitro thrombelastography study. Br J Anaesth 78:684–689

35. A report by the American Society of Anesthesiologists Task Force on Blood Component Therapy (1996) Practice guidelines for blood component therapy. Anesthesiology 84:732–747

36. Looker D, Abbott-Brown D, Cozart P, Durfee S, Hoffman S, Mathews AJ, Miller-Roerich J, Shoemaker S, Trimble S, Fermi G, Komiyama NH, Nagai K, Stetler GL (1992) A human recombinant haemoglobin designed for use as a blood substitute. Nature 356:258–260

37. Dieryck W, Pagnier J, Poyart C, Marden MC, Gruber V, Bournat P, Baudino S, Merot B (1997) Human haemoglobin from transgenic tobacco. Nature 386:29–30

Subject Index

A

abdominal surgery 8
acarbia 27
acid-base regulation 104
acidosis 37, 123
– lactic 123
– metabolic 37
adhesion molecules 52, 53, 70
a-adrenergic receptors 125
AIS (abbreviated injury score) 30
albumin 1–22
– albumin levels in critical illness 3, 4
– consensus recommendations 8
– hypoalbuminaemia, clinical outcome 4, 5
– perioperative volume replacement, albumin supplementation 7, 8
– physiological characteristics 2
– shock resuscitation (see also shock) 5–7
allergic/anaphylactoid reactions 15, 50, 60, 63, 68, 108

AMI (acute myocardial infarction) 39, 40
amylase 126
amylase 48, 126
– a-amylases 77
anaesthetic agents 38
angioplasty 40
antibodies
– against HES 15
– antidextran 16
– dextran-reactive 63
antithrombotic effects 13, 60
anuria 37, 114
– oligoanuria 115
aortic surgery 8
ARDS (adult respiratory distress syndrome) 8, 28, 31, 32, 36
– major burns 31, 32
L-arginine 125
artificial colloids 1, 14
ATLS (advanced trauma life support) 28
atrial natriuretic peptide (ANP) 69
autologous blood 124

Springer
and the
environment

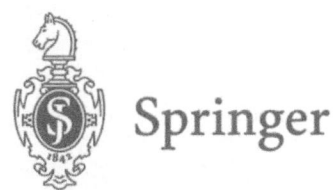

Springer